healthy eating
to reduce the risk
of dementia

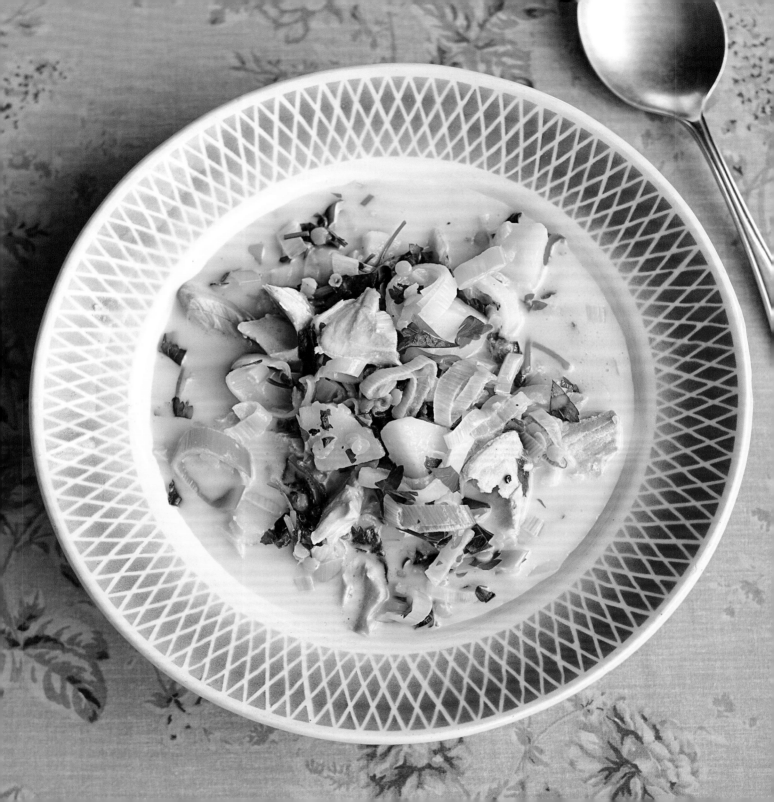

Margaret Rayman BSc, DPhil (Oxon), RNutr,
Katie Sharpe BSc, RD,
Vanessa Ridland BSc, RD
& Patsy Westcott BA, MSc (Nutr Med)

University of Surrey

healthy eating
to reduce the risk
of dementia

100 fantastic recipes based on extensive, in-depth research

Photography by Will Heap

Kyle Books

An Hachette UK Company
www.hachette.co.uk

First published in Great Britain in 2015 by
Kyle Books, an imprint of Kyle Cathie Ltd
Carmelite House
50 Victoria Embankment
London EC4Y 0DZ
www.kylebooks.co.uk

This edition published in 2019

ISBN 978 0 85783 753 0

Distributed in the US by Hachette Book Group,
1290 Avenue of the Americas, 4th and 5th Floors,
New York, NY 10104

Distributed in Canada by Canadian Manda Group,
664 Annette St., Toronto, Ontario, Canada M6S 2C8

Project Editor: Tara O'Sullivan
Copy Editor: Clare Sayer
Designer: Arno Devo
Illustrations: Arno Devo*
Photographer: Will Heap
Food Stylist: Annie Nichols**
Prop Stylist: Iris Bromet
Production: Nic Jones and Gemma John
*Except Mediterranean Diet Pyramid, page 36. Illustration
by George Middleton, © Oldways Preservation and
Exchange Trust
**Except pages 42, 45, 49, 57, 75, 77, 81, 86, 125, 139,
152, 156 & 159, Rachel Wood

Printed and bound in China

10 9 8 7 6 5 4 3 2 1

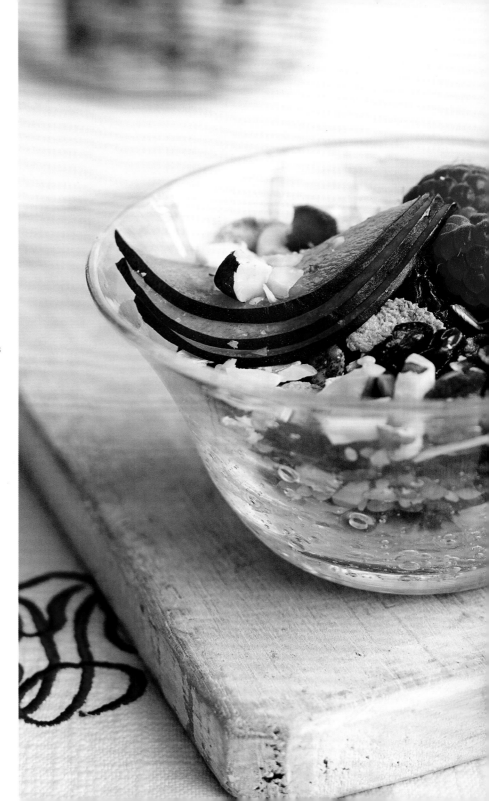

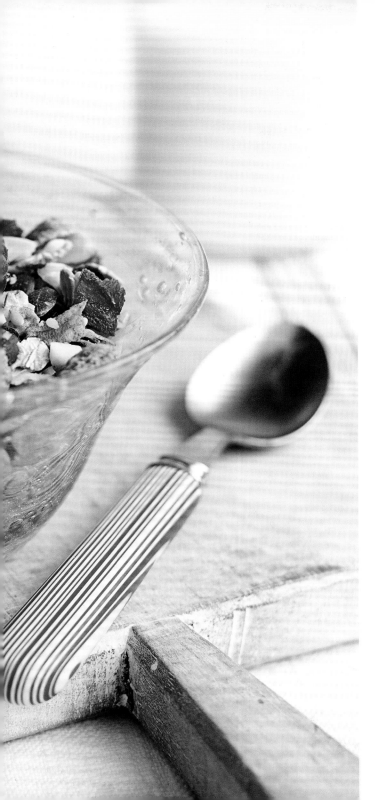

contents

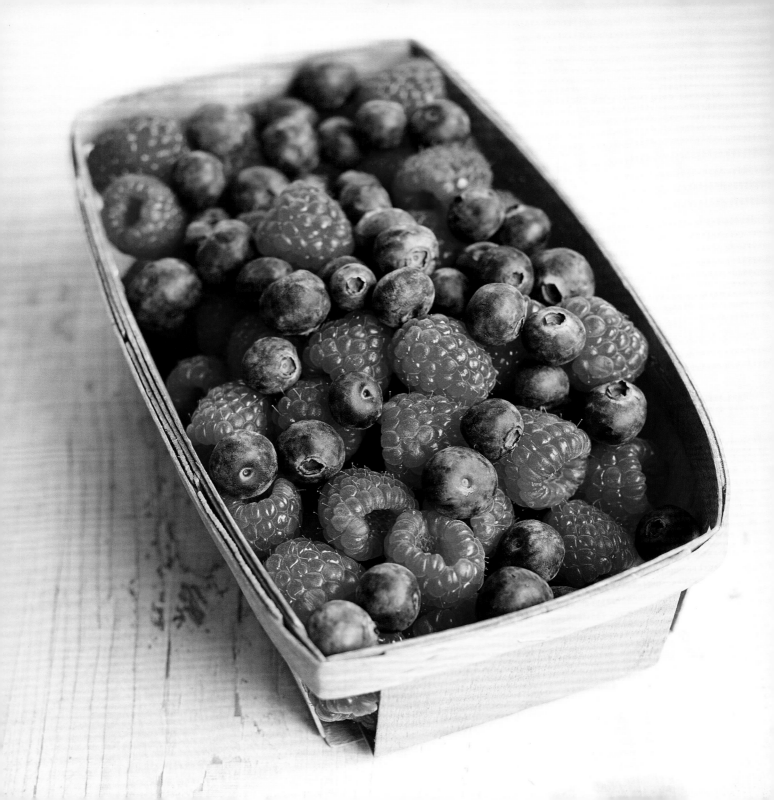

foreword

One of the things we notice as we get older is that our memory does not seem to be as good as it used to be. There is indeed evidence from many cross-sectional studies comparing old and young that some cognitive abilities are impaired in the elderly but, on the other hand, up to about the age of 60 other cognitive abilities actually improve due to greater experience. Change in the population as a whole is called "usual aging." Some scientists have suggested that "usual brain aging" in a population is a mixture of "disease-related aging" in some people and "successful brain aging" in others. Among the factors that help to maintain "successful brain aging" is control of high blood pressure, prevention of diabetes and regular exercise. This welcome book looks at whether nutrition also plays a role in successful brain aging. When you hear reports in the media about diet and the brain and wonder whether they are true or not, then look for the answers here.

Hardly a week goes by without some report in the press about how a certain diet can protect you against getting Alzheimer's disease, or against memory decline. These reports are usually based upon a single scientific paper and they are often exaggerated so the reader is left uncertain about what to do. This situation is partly because nutritional science is not as straightforward as some of the other sciences. We eat food, not a mixture of pure vitamins or minerals. Scientists want to identify which components of food are crucial for brain function and so they do clinical trials in which pure components of food are given to people for many months and carry out memory tests before and after the treatment. These trials do not always work as expected and so we need to look at particular foods and at dietary patterns as well as at pure chemicals. A well-known example is the Mediterranean diet, which is complex and not easy to define in chemical terms.

Memory decline may be relatively trivial or it may be an early part of a process that eventually leads to Alzheimer's disease. This develops slowly, over 20 to 30 years, and it is only in the last five to ten years that we begin to notice memory problems. The long gestation of the disease provides an opportunity to modify the disease process and so to prevent dementia. Our genes play a role in that some of them increase the risk that we will develop dementia but only very rarely indeed do they make it inevitable that we will get the disease. For most people who develop dementia, the causes are multiple and risk-factor genes are just one component. We now believe that nutritional factors also play a role and that they interact with each other and with the risk-factor genes. As we age, some of the components of our diet essential for brain function are not as well absorbed as when we were younger, for example vitamin B12. We need to be aware of this and eat the right kind of foods or even take a vitamin supplement. So it is a complicated story and you need a book like this to help you. As well as telling you about the science in a very clear and balanced way, the book encourages you to put into practice what we already know by providing a range of recipes. So, go for it—and help yourself and your brain to age successfully!

A. DAVID SMITH FMEDSCI
Professor Emeritus of Pharmacology, University of Oxford

Professor Smith co-founded the Oxford Project to Investigate Memory and Ageing in 1988. In 1998 OPTIMA identified raised plasma homocysteine and low-normal folate and vitamin B12 as risk factors for Alzheimer's disease and in 2009 OPTIMA completed a successful clinical trial of B vitamin supplements in people with Mild Cognitive Impairment.

Introduction Diet and dementia

Dementia, including Alzheimer's disease (AD), is a major and growing health problem all over the world. Most of our lives are touched by it, and many of us will have relatives, friends, colleagues or acquaintances who are affected. In 2013 there were more than 44 million people with dementia worldwide and by 2050 there will be 135 million. Meanwhile, in the UK, according to the Alzheimer's Society, around 800,000 people are living with dementia, a figure set to rise to over a million by 2021. And, although a handful of drugs can help control initial symptoms and may slow its progress, there is currently no cure.

The financial cost of dementia globally is a staggering $530 billion, while in the UK the NHS, local authorities and families spend around £23 billion ($30 billion) per year— twice as much as on cancer, three times as much as on heart disease and four times as much as on stroke. But this is small compared to the incalculable emotional, physical and psychological strain dementia places on those who have it, their families and friends.

Age is the biggest risk factor for dementia. Around one in 100 people aged 60 to 64 years has some form of it, while by age 95 one in three people is affected. Despite this, dementia is not inevitable. There are things you can do to help reduce your risk. Simple lifestyle measures such as staying physically active, not smoking, watching your weight, keeping an eye on your cholesterol and blood pressure and, above all, eating a healthy diet may help to protect your brain and keep it sharp as you age.

Scarcely a week passes without some dramatic news item about the miraculous effects of this or that food or nutrient on brain health. Sadly, many are overblown and inaccurate. Despite the headlines, research—including research into nutrition—rarely progresses in a straight line. Instead, evidence accumulates bit by bit until it is too strong to ignore.

In this book we look beyond the hype to bring you reliable, up-to-date advice, based on the latest scientific research, about the foods and nutrients most likely to protect your brain and help reduce your risk of dementia. To this end we trawled though numerous studies on diet and nutrition and assessed the quality of their evidence.

As we researched, two things became clear. One is that the whole is greater than the parts. A diet high in fresh fruit and vegetables, whole grains, pulses, fish, nuts, seeds and oils such as olive oil, but low in saturated and trans-fats and processed foods, is likely to provide you with the best combination of nutrients in the optimal amounts to help protect your brain.

The other is that, for the most part, a healthy, varied diet is likely to benefit your brain and offer better protection from cognitive decline and dementia than taking isolated nutrients as supplements.

In this book you will learn more about the nutrients, foods and dietary patterns that make for a healthy brain, as well as how to incorporate them into your lifestyle. To help you put our findings into practice we have devised more than 100 delicious recipes that we hope will help you to choose the foods most likely to lower your risk of developing dementia and enable you to adapt your own favorite dishes.

There are no easy solutions to dementia. We cannot guarantee that you can or will avoid it. And we certainly do not promise a cure. But, we do believe that making some simple, sustainable dietary choices can help to protect the health of your brain.

Enjoy!

FOOD SYNERGY

Although many studies strongly suggest a relationship between what we eat and long-term brain health, the picture is confused and confusing. Researchers are increasingly looking at "food synergy," the idea that, although the effects of single foods or nutrients may be small, when you combine them in a healthy diet they can pack a powerful punch. In particular a Mediterranean style of eating is associated with longer life expectancy and lower rates of chronic diseases, including dementia. See page 36.

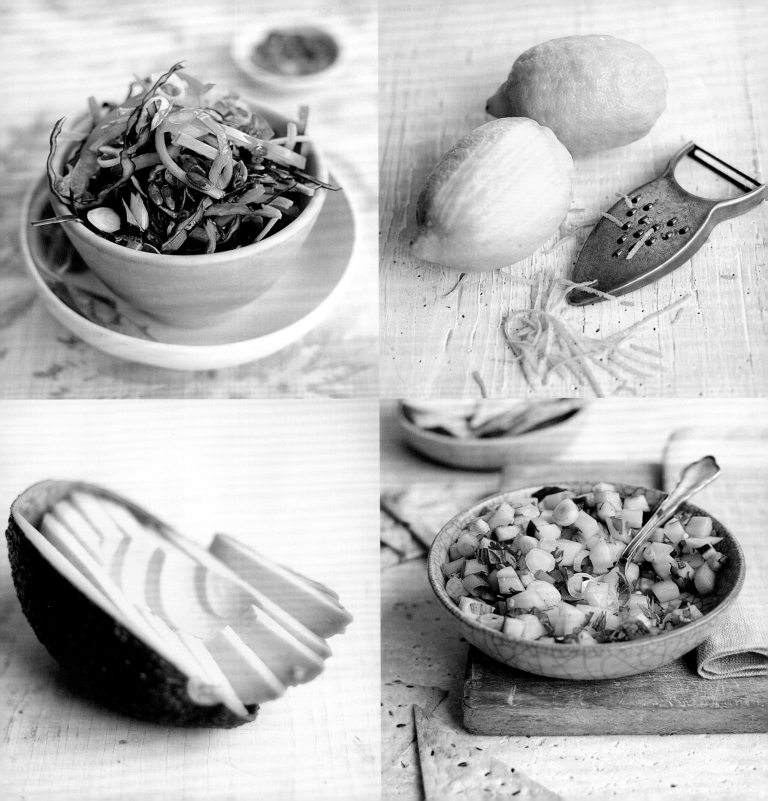

Making sense of dietary research

Before reading what you can do to help keep your brain healthy, it will help to understand a bit about dietary research and how it is carried out.

Until recently, research into brain aging and neurodegenerative disease was relatively poorly funded. This is slowly changing and new findings are appearing more often. These findings can be conflicting and not always easy to interpret, however, and all too often, and most frustratingly, the conclusion is "more research is needed." We haven't shied away from reporting negative or contradictory results, but we have tried to put them into context to help you make up your own mind.

Several different types of studies are used to examine how foods, nutrients or patterns of eating may affect the risk of disease, each of which has strengths and weaknesses. Some are performed in laboratories, some are conducted on animals and others are carried out on people. But while findings from the former can help identify underlying mechanisms, they don't necessarily translate to humans. And human studies can be equally fraught with difficulties, for reasons including:

- lack of a foolproof way to gather accurate information about food intake in groups of people
- difficulty assessing whether people are eating what they say they are
- similar foods can have different nutritional profiles depending on how and where they are grown
- gaps in our knowledge about the precise nutrient content of many foods
- not knowing whether low blood levels of nutrients in people with Alzheimer's disease are a cause or consequence of the disease process.

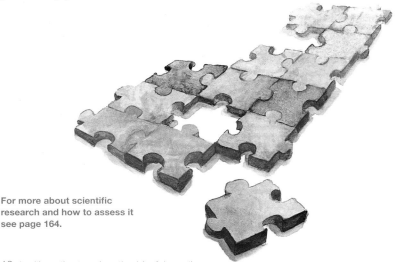

For more about scientific research and how to assess it see page 164.

Types of study

One way to reduce the margin of error and compensate for inaccuracy is to gather information from large numbers of people in randomized controlled trials (RCTs) that are more likely to prove cause and effect (see Appendix 2). Most evidence linking diet and dementia, however, comes from studies that draw inferences about the effects of foods, nutrients or eating patterns on groups of people by observing them over time. These observational studies can help researchers develop ideas about how certain foods and nutrients are associated with disease, but they cannot prove cause and effect.

What they can do is identify potentially beneficial nutrients, foods and dietary patterns. When lots of such studies involving thousands of participants from different places reach the same or similar conclusions—and when there is convincing evidence to explain how they may work—they can provide a basis for cautious dietary recommendations. This makes even more sense if the recommendations are safe, easy to follow and have other health benefits. This is the approach we take in this book.

Until recently, although there were clues, few parts of the diet and dementia puzzle fitted. Now more pieces have been added and we are getting a better idea of the whole picture. Some pieces are still missing, however, and others may be in the wrong place. It is likely to take years to complete the puzzle. Meanwhile, there are positive steps you can take right now to help protect your brain against dementia.

About dementia

Dementia is a set of symptoms caused by several different diseases that affect the brain. Symptoms vary but include memory loss, problems with thinking (impaired cognition), mood changes and loss of coordination.

Alzheimer's disease

Alzheimer's disease (AD), which affects 62 percent of people with dementia, is the leading cause of dementia. It has two key hallmarks—the formation of microscopic clusters or plaques of a protein known as amyloid-beta (Aβ) in the brain, and the build-up of twisted strands of another protein called tau, known as neurofibrillary tangles, both of which are toxic to the brain.

Over time the connections between brain cells (synapses) dwindle, stopping brain cells communicating with each other. Eventually the damage becomes so great that brain cells die and regions such as the hippocampus, which is concerned with memory and learning, shrink—a process called brain atrophy.

It is not known exactly what causes all this to happen but recently inflammation and insulin resistance—when the body is unable to use insulin properly—have been recognized as key players in the development of AD. Whatever the cause, the brain changes that lead to the disease start 20 to 30 years before symptoms become apparent, meaning that there is a window of time during which it may be possible to slow down the process and protect the brain.

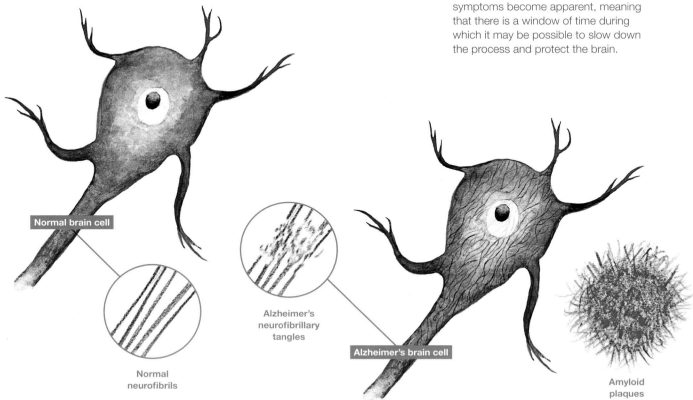

Normal brain cell

Normal neurofibrils

Alzheimer's neurofibrillary tangles

Alzheimer's brain cell

Amyloid plaques

Vascular dementia

Caused by problems with the brain's blood supply, vascular dementia affects 17 percent of people with the disease. It happens when less oxygen reaches the brain due to narrowed or blocked blood vessels. This in turn damages brain cells or causes their death. Vascular dementia can develop rapidly after a stroke or, more gradually, as a result of ongoing blood-vessel damage.

Mixed and other dementias

Dementia caused by both Alzheimer's disease and vascular or other forms of dementia is known as "mixed dementia," meaning that the symptoms have more than one cause. Rarer forms of dementia make up a small percentage of cases and dementia can also be a symptom of other conditions, such as Parkinson's disease.

Mild Cognitive Impairment

Mild cognitive impairment (MCI) affects 3–19 percent of over 65-year-olds. People with it often have problems with memory or thinking, but these do not significantly interfere with everyday life. MCI is not dementia and may remain stable or even return to normal. However, it does increase the risk of dementia and an estimated 10–15 percent of those with it develop dementia each year.

THE GENETIC CONNECTION

Several genes have been linked to an increased risk of dementia. The most studied are versions (variants) of the ApoE gene, which enables fats to be carried around the bloodstream and delivered to cells. The ApoE ε2 version is linked to a lower risk of AD. The ApoE ε4 version is linked to a higher risk of late-onset AD, the kind that develops after age 65. Only half of people with AD have the ApoE ε4 gene, however, reflecting the many other factors involved in AD.

RISK FACTORS FOR DEMENTIA

Some you cannot do anything about:
Age—The older you are, the greater your risk.
Genes—Some genes are associated with a greater or lesser risk of dementia.
Gender—Women are more at risk of AD. Although is not yet known why, it is not just because women live longer than men.

Some you can modify:
Risk factors for heart disease and stroke—High cholesterol, high blood pressure, overweight, high blood glucose levels and type-2 diabetes all increase the risk of dementia and AD—so looking after your heart can help protect your brain.

Physical activity—Being physically active can help reduce the risk of cognitive decline and dementia and research suggests that it works in synergy with nutrients to help protect the brain.
Smoking—Smoking increases the risk of vascular dementia and vascular aspects of Alzheimer's disease. This risk goes down within two to four years of stopping smoking.
Diet—As you will see throughout this book, paying attention to what you eat is one of the things you can do yourself to help protect your brain against dementia.

The brain-protective diet

Antioxidants in the brain-protective diet

The antioxidant vitamins A, C, E and beta-carotene, together with the mineral selenium, help to keep us healthy in body and mind. Many scientists speculate that we need more antioxidants as we get older to combat cell damage caused by oxidative stress (see box on the right), now thought to be a driving force behind many chronic diseases, including Alzheimer's disease and vascular dementia. People with AD and dementia have fewer antioxidants in their blood than healthy people, although whether this is a cause or a consequence of the disease is not known.

Emerging evidence suggests that dietary antioxidants are likely to work in synergy. Including a combination of foods such as fruit, vegetables, nuts and seeds that are rich in vitamins E and C, the most studied in relation to brain and vascular health, as well as other beneficial vitamins, minerals, plant compounds and fiber is likely to have the best long-term benefits for your brain.

What is the evidence?

In laboratory and animal studies vitamins E and C block the cascade of damage triggered by molecules called reactive oxygen species. There is also evidence that they can reduce the vascular damage that increases the risk of heart and brain problems. However, despite their apparent promise, it has proved frustratingly difficult to show definite benefits.

In 2004 researchers from the Taub Institute for Research on Alzheimer's Disease and the Aging Brain at Columbia University in the US examined seven studies looking at the potential links between antioxidant intake and the risk of dementia and Alzheimer's disease. In all but one, higher intakes of vitamin C and/or vitamin E were associated with a lower risk of AD and/or dementia—especially when obtained from the diet. But not all studies are positive. For example, one study of almost 3,000 older people carried out in 2008 found no reduced risk for either Alzheimer's disease or dementia when participants took supplementary vitamins E and C. The picture is unclear. However, one common theme is that getting your antioxidants in food appears to be more effective than taking them as supplements.

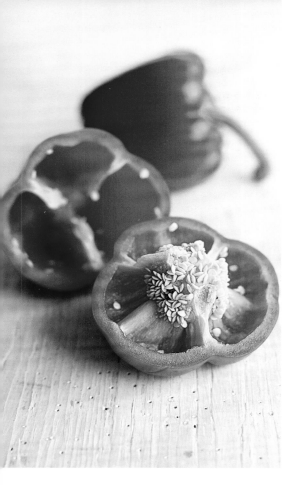

Know your antioxidants

Vitamin C

Vitamin C (ascorbate) is a water-soluble antioxidant. One of its major roles is to mop up free radicals. Because it dissolves in water it is not stored in the body, so you need to consume vitamin C-rich foods every day to ensure good levels in your bloodstream.

Food sources

Most fruits and vegetables contain vitamin C. Blackcurrants, kiwis, citrus fruit and raw peppers are some of the best sources, but even the humble potato can add to your daily intake. In fact, potatoes and potato products contribute more vitamin C to the UK diet than any other food.

Because it is water-soluble, vitamin C is easily lost in cooking water and can be destroyed by high heat. Cooking methods such as steaming or stir-frying can help minimize losses, as can putting vegetables in casseroles. Be sure too to eat plenty of fresh, uncooked fruit and vegetables to make the most of vitamin C.

What is the evidence?

Some studies suggest that regular consumption of 80–250 milligrams a day (which should be from food rather than supplements) may be optimum for cognitive function, but researchers all agree that one of the most vital roles for this vitamin is to support the antioxidant activities of vitamin E (see opposite).

How does it work?

Many antioxidants work both together and alone to exert their effects. So, for example, vitamin C can enhance the action of vitamin E. Specifically, vitamin C works by:

- scavenging free radicals in the blood and inside cells
- helping to recycle vitamin E so it keeps on working
- increasing the total amount of antioxidants that can be stored and used in our tissues
- stabilizing other chemicals in blood and cells to keep blood vessels healthy.

Are we getting enough?

The amount of vitamin C needed for optimal health is unknown. However, it has been suggested that in older people and smokers, who are at high risk of oxidative stress, intakes may be too low. In the UK the recommended intake for adults is 40 milligrams a day; however, other countries recommend more: 75 milligrams a day in the US, for example. There is much debate among scientists about whether recommended amounts should be increased, especially for groups at high risk of oxidative damage.

Recommendations

Ways to ensure you get plenty of vitamin C include:

- eating plenty of raw or lightly cooked fruit and vegetables daily—citrus fruits, berries and peppers are all good sources
- smokers, the elderly and other at-risk groups might want to consider taking a modest supplement.

NB The amount of vitamin C in general multivitamin and mineral supplements sold over the counter should be safe.

However, avoid doubling up on vitamin supplements to prevent overdosing.

Points to note

- At low intakes, we absorb vitamin C efficiently but at high intakes (more than 1.5 grams a day) we absorb little.
- High-dose supplements of vitamin C (>2g/day) may cause abdominal discomfort and/or diarrhoea.
- If long-term supplementation is stopped suddenly, some people may show symptoms of scurvy.

Vitamin E

Although vitamin E is often thought of as just one nutrient, there are in fact eight different fat-soluble forms. The two main ones are alpha- and gamma-tocopherol. Until recently, alpha-tocopherol was thought to be the most biologically active, but it is now thought other forms may be equally important for health. As well as its antioxidant activity, vitamin E may play a role in brain health by helping to dampen down inflammation and prevent the production of potentially damaging inflammatory chemicals. In animal and laboratory investigations, gamma-tocopherol has been found to be a more potent anti-inflammatory than alpha-tocopherol. It also appears to be more efficient at scavenging certain free radicals. Vitamin E has been much studied in relation to heart disease and a high dietary intake has also been linked to a reduced risk of some cancers (prostate, colorectal, lung and esophageal).

Food sources

Vegetable oils, wheatgerm, nuts (especially almonds, Brazil nuts and

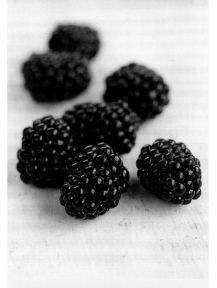

SOURCES OF GAMMA-TOCOPHEROL

Gamma-tocopherol has potent anti-inflammatory effects and can remove damaging chemicals known as reactive nitrogen species (RNS). Good sources include:
- Canola oil
- Wheatgerm
- Pecan nuts
- Cashews
- Brazil nuts
- Walnuts
- Peanuts
- Sesame seeds
- Blackberries

pecans) and seeds (particularly sunflower and sesame) all contain vitamin E, as do cereals and cereal products. Alpha-tocopherol is the main source of vitamin E in the UK due to its presence in sunflower oil, which is much used in cooking and food-processing. In the US, where corn oil is more widely used, gamma-tocopherol is the main form.

Dark green leafy vegetables such as kale, watercress and spinach also contain some vitamin E, with smaller quantities found in some beans and pulses. Avocados, blackberries and salmon contain moderate amounts and egg yolks a small amount.

Fish such as tuna and sardines that have been canned in oil containing vitamin E can contribute a small amount to intake. Bought salad dressings, spreads, cookies, pastries and other baked goods also contain vitamin E as vegetable oils are often used in their production. However, they can be high in calories, sugar, salt and saturated fat and low in beneficial nutrients, so are not the best source.

What is the evidence?

Vitamin E has been much studied in relation to dementia, with mixed results. For example, a large European study published in 2010, with almost 6,000 participants, found that those who obtained the most vitamin E from food (18.5 milligrams a day) were 25 percent less likely to develop dementia than those with low-to-moderate intakes (9–13.5 milligrams a day). Similar results were reported for the risk of AD. In 2005, when over 1,000 men and women over 65 were assessed over a six-year period, researchers found that there was a 25 percent reduction in risk for every 5 milligrams a day by which alpha- and gamma-tocopherol from the diet increased. The benefits of high dietary (rather than supplemental) intakes strongly suggest that a combination of different tocopherols may be most effective in maintaining brain health. This finding is supported by several reviews of evidence confirming that vitamin E forms other than alpha-tocopherol may be beneficial and that vitamin E supplements—generally alpha-tocopherol—are unlikely to be

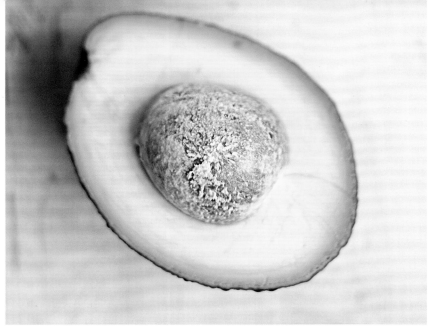

- Do not take a vitamin E supplement if you have a clotting disorder or are taking anticoagulant medication, such as warfarin.
- Avoid high-dose supplements (more than 200 IU or 133 milligrams a day).
- Prolonged high doses may increase your risk of haemorrhagic stroke, caused by rupture of a blood vessel in the brain.
- In an RCT, a supplement of 400 IU alpha-tocopherol a day increased the risk of prostate cancer by 17 percent.
- Taking a standard over-the-counter (OTC) multivitamin product is known to be safe and will not provide excess amounts of either vitamin C or vitamin E.

protective against Alzheimer's disease, dementia, vascular or heart disease.

One thing is clear: most research suggests that getting your vitamin E from food rather than supplements is more likely to protect your brain.

How does it work?
Vitamin E:
- breaks the chain of oxidative damage set off by free radicals
- works in the blood vessels to prevent the first step toward atherosclerosis
- has other effects that may reduce cell aging and neurodegeneration
- works alone and with vitamin C to help protect against oxidative stress and cell damage
- has other protective functions. Along with vitamin C, it can slow the production of enzymes and other chemicals that could reduce the efficiency of blood circulation. They both also reduce inflammation in several systems in the body.

Are we getting enough?
Although there is no recommended intake, in the UK men consume around 10.6 milligrams and women around 8.1 milligrams of vitamin E a day. The amount needed to maintain good antioxidant status is thought to depend on the amount of polyunsaturated fats (PUFAs) in your diet. The more PUFAs you consume, the more are stored in your body and the more vitamin E you need to protect them from oxidation. Deficiency is rare, although consuming a very low-fat diet, which is likely to be low in vitamin E, may put you at risk.

Recommendations
Easy ways to maximize your intake of the different forms of vitamin E include:
- using canola oil (which has good levels of gamma- as well as alpha-tocopherol) for cooking
- sprinkling wheatgerm on your breakfast cereal
- snacking on almonds, pecans or sunflower seeds.

VITAMIN E AND THE VASCULAR SYSTEM

Vitamin E appears to be especially important for the health of the blood vessels and circulation, which are vital for a healthy brain. A large review of almost 50 studies, which included an analysis of the vitamin E intake of over a million men and women, found that those with the highest intake from food and/or higher levels in their blood, which reflects dietary intake, had a lower risk of problems such as heart attacks and strokes. By contrast, taking a vitamin E supplement did not improve blood vessel health.

Selenium

Selenium, a trace mineral found in soil, is known for its antioxidant effects and other benefits. Though we only need small amounts, according to several studies it may help protect against dementia. In fact, it is so important for a healthy brain that, if the diet lacks selenium, the brain conserves it at the expense of other tissues. Studies also show that selenium deficiency causes irreversible brain damage—at least in a study looking at mice.

Food sources
Selenium levels in food vary from country to country. In North America, which has selenium-rich soil, bread and cereals are the main source. In the UK and Europe, where soil levels are lower, meat and poultry are key sources. Brazil nuts are the richest food source but they also contain barium and radium, which may damage health, so be careful not to overindulge. Offal, especially kidney, fish and seafood are other good sources (see Appendix 3).

What is the evidence?
Animal and laboratory studies suggest that selenium may help prevent brain cells from dying by preventing Alzheimer's plaques and tangles from forming. There are fewer human studies; however, one, which measured selenium levels in the blood of people with mild AD, showed that they had significantly lower selenium concentrations than a comparable group of healthy people. As with other nutrients, it is not known whether this was a cause or an effect of the disease.

Some of the most persuasive evidence that selenium may protect the brain comes from a long-running study of older inhabitants of Nantes in western France. In a group of 1,166 people with healthy brains at the outset, those with low blood levels of selenium were more likely to show signs of cognitive decline four years later. Nine years on from the start of the study, those with the steepest fall in selenium levels had the largest decline in cognitive function.

As with other nutrients, not all research on selenium and dementia points the same way. A study of 4,809 Americans carried out as part of the US government's third national nutrition survey, for example, found no association between memory and blood levels of selenium. By contrast, among 2,000 rural Chinese people aged over 65, those with the lowest levels of selenium in their toenails (a good way to measure selenium), scored lower in four out of five tests of cognitive function.

One small but encouraging clinical trial has examined the effects of selenium as a sole nutrient. Thirty people with Alzheimer's disease were assigned to take either 100 micrograms of organic selenium or a placebo every other day in ten three-week cycles over the course of a year. At the end of this time, the condition of 13 of the 15 taking selenium had stabilized, compared to only eight of the 16 who took the placebo.

How does it work?
Many selenoproteins, a family of proteins with selenium at their core, are antioxidant enzymes. Two selenoproteins in particular may be especially important in protecting the brain:

- **Selenoprotein M**, which in animal studies reduces Aβ production and protects brain function.
- **Selenoprotein P**, which appears to have a special role in delivering selenium to the brain—by latching on to a receptor on the surface of brain cells rather like a key in a lock. In the laboratory, it helps neurons to survive oxidative stress caused by Aβ. The nerve cells of mice that cannot synthesize selenoprotein P are more likely to degenerate, leading to tight, stiff muscles, abnormal movements and spontaneous seizures.

Are we getting enough?
Official recommendations for selenium intake vary around the world but average 60 micrograms a day (men) and 53 micrograms a day (women). Intakes are high in Venezuela, Canada, the USA and Japan and lower in the UK and Europe, especially Eastern Europe. In China intakes range from very low to very high. In Europe, the average intake is around 40 micrograms a day. In the US, it is around 95 micrograms a day (women) and 135 micrograms a day (men). Selenium supplements are popular, especially in the US, where some 50 percent of people take dietary supplements.

Supplementary benefits
Getting enough selenium is important not just for your brain but also for immune function, greater resistance to viruses and a lower risk of autoimmune thyroid disease. Selenium is also essential for fertility in both men and women. Higher selenium levels may

also help reduce the risk of prostate, lung, bowel and bladder cancers according to observational studies, although findings from clinical trials have been mixed. This may be because, as with other nutrients, supplementation is only likely to benefit those with inadequate intake.

Recommendations

- If you live in a part of the world such as the UK or Europe where intakes are less than 60 micrograms a day (men) or 53 micrograms a day (women), try to include good sources of selenium, such as kidneys, liver, fish, shellfish and occasionally Brazil nuts, in your diet.
- If you never eat these foods, go for a low-dose selenium supplement of 50–100 micrograms a day, maximum.
- Multivitamin and mineral supplements often contain selenium. Check the label and if it contains 30–50 micrograms, that is sufficient.

Point to note

Extra selenium may benefit you if you have a low intake of selenium. If you have an adequate-to-high intake (e.g. you live in North America, Venezuela, Japan or some parts of China) do not take a selenium supplement; it could increase the risk of health problems such as non-melanoma skin cancer and type-2 diabetes.

Polyphenols in the brain-protective diet

Polyphenols are naturally occurring chemicals produced by plants to deter pests, protect against disease and defend against UV damage. The bitter flavor of coffee, the astringent aftertaste of certain red wines, the deep blue and purple of blueberries and eggplants, and the rich scent of vanilla all stem from polyphenols.

Polyphenols can help protect against heart disease, certain cancers, diabetes and high blood pressure. There is also increasing evidence that they may reduce the risk of dementia and AD. Foods rich in polyphenols also often contain other beneficial nutrients such as vitamins, minerals and fiber, as well as being generally low in calories. We still have much to learn about polyphenols and how they work but it is clear that we need to include plenty of polyphenol-rich foods in our daily diet.

Food sources

Scientists have identified more than 8,000 polyphenols, of which around 200 are consumed in the diet. Widely found in fruit, vegetables, peas, beans and lentils, cereals and drinks, the ones most studied for their brain benefits include those in cocoa, red wine, grapes, berries, citrus fruits, soy products, coffee and green and black tea.

What is the evidence?

Extensive evidence from animal studies shows that polyphenols in cocoa, wine, grapes and berries can improve memory and learning. In other studies, polyphenols from the flesh and skin of citrus fruits have been found to slow the formation of tau protein tangles.

Consumption of red wine, vegetable and fruit juices has been found to delay the onset of dementia and/or Alzheimer's disease. These benefits may be most marked in carriers of the ApoE ε4 gene variant, as well as in smokers and the physically inactive, according to a study of Japanese-Americans.

A French study revealed that people with a high intake of polyphenols had a smaller decline in brain function over a ten-year period. A 2013 review of 16 clinical studies, meanwhile, confirmed that a diet high in fruit and vegetables was linked to healthier blood circulation and lower blood pressure, both of which can contribute to brain health. In this review, beet—the deep-purple color reflects its polyphenol content—was especially beneficial.

How do they work?

Polyphenols may act in several different ways including:
- as antioxidants
- as anti-inflammatory factors
- preventing deterioration in brain cells
- improving blood flow to the brain
- helping to maintain stable blood glucose levels—this can reduce damage to blood vessels in the brain
- improving brain function—some flavonoids may act on specific brain regions to improve memory and learning and even stimulate new protein production and new connections between brain cells.

Are we getting enough?

Unlike traditional vitamins, polyphenols are not essential to day-to-day health

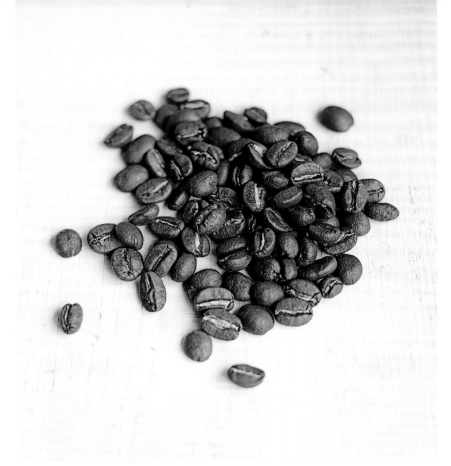

- Drinking up to six cups a day of black or green tea, three to four cups of coffee and one or two small glasses of red wine a day could have benefits.
- Herbs and spices are rich in polyphenols and an excellent way to add flavor and extra beneficial nutrients.
- Include soy foods such as soybeans, soy milk, tofu and tempeh in your diet several times a week.
- Regularly eating moderate amounts of nuts, particularly pistachios, will also help to keep your blood vessels healthy.

Points to note
- Drinking too much alcohol increases the risk of many chronic diseases, so keep your intake of red wine within safe limits (see page 38).
- If you don't drink, simply choose polyphenols from other sources such as grapes and berries.

and there is no recommended intake. Estimating how many of the different polyphenols we consume can be difficult, but in the UK, average total intake is probably around 780 milligrams a day (women) and 1,000 milligrams a day (men), although some people may be getting as little as 30 milligrams and others as much as 2,300 milligrams a day.

Recommendations
- Polyphenols and their products in the body may not be stored for long in the bloodstream. The best way to ensure a steady supply is to include a wide variety of different polyphenol-containing foods in your daily diet.
- Aim for between five and nine 80-gram (3-ounce) portions of fruit and vegetables a day—opt for apples, onions, eggplants, berry fruits, beet, carrots, citrus fruit (including zest and/or pith), grapes, apricots, cruciferous vegetables (such as broccoli, red and green cabbage, kale, watercress) and tomatoes.

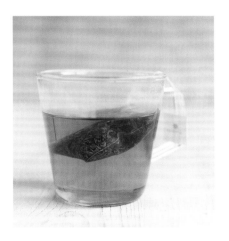

FOODS AND DRINKS CONTAINING POLYPHENOLS OF PARTICULAR RELEVANCE TO BRAIN HEALTH INCLUDE:

Red wine and grapes
A moderate intake of red wine has been linked with a lower risk of dementia. Resveratrol, a polyphenol found in red wine and also in grape juice, may be the active ingredient. In fruit flies and small mammals, resveratrol can extend life by several hundred percent although there are, as yet, no effective human studies. Grape polyphenols may also help reduce the formation of Aβ plaques and tau tangles.

Soy products
Soy products contain polyphenols called isoflavones, which, in some small studies, have been found to improve short- and long-term memory, mental flexibility and decision-making. One such study, carried out in Japan, found that regular, moderate consumption of tofu and tempeh, a product made from fermented soybeans, was linked to better immediate recall, although benefits applied only to those aged 67 or younger. A high intake of soybeans and soy products as part of a "Japanese dietary pattern" has also been associated with a significantly reduced risk of all forms of dementia.

Tea and coffee
Some studies into the effects of drinking green and black tea and coffee on dementia or AD risk have found a significant protective effect, although results have been inconsistent.

Pistachio nuts
Pistachio nuts are rich in several polyphenols as well as gamma-tocopherol, vitamin C, beta-carotene and selenium. One or two servings of pistachios a day (a serving is 30–60 grams/1–2 ounces) was shown to increase antioxidants in the blood. They also prevented "bad" LDL cholesterol from becoming damaged, a key trigger for atherosclerosis in adults with high cholesterol. They also lowered blood pressure in people with high levels of blood fats.

Cocoa and chocolate
Polyphenols called flavanols found in cocoa and bittersweet chocolate may be especially beneficial to brain health. According to more than 20 clinical trials, they reduce many risk factors for dementia in both healthy people and those with circulatory problems. Benefits include lower blood pressure, improved blood flow to the brain and enhanced flexibility of blood vessels. Cocoa flavanols can also reduce blood stickiness and may improve insulin resistance, which is linked to type-2 diabetes and a higher risk of dementia.

Citrus fruits
Drinking either grapefruit or orange juice every day can reduce blood pressure and improve the health of blood vessels, according to a 2013 review. Similar results were found when the citrus polyphenol hesperidin was tested against a placebo.

Another study found that consuming 750 milliliters (3 cups) of orange juice daily increased "good" HDL cholesterol, reduced blood fats and decreased the ratio of "bad" LDL to "good" HDL cholesterol in people with high cholesterol. Although drinking this amount of juice is not a good idea because of its high calorie and sugar content, eating whole citrus fruits or using them in cooking could help you reap the benefits.

Berries
Blueberries, blackberries, cherries, raspberries and other purple and dark red berries are rich in polyphenols called anthocyanins. Numerous animal studies have shown that these can improve many aspects of brain function and may even stimulate the growth of new brain cells. In 2012, for instance, researchers reported that in a group of over 16,000 older people who regularly ate blueberries and strawberries, cognitive decline was delayed by up to 2.5 years.

Berry polyphenols may also help the brain to stay healthy through their effects on vascular health. A daily intake of anthocyanins over six to eight weeks has been shown to reduce blood pressure in people with risk factors for heart disease and those who have had a heart attack. Similar benefits have been shown with long-term consumption (3–18 months) of pomegranate juice— all good reasons to put berries and pomegranates on the menu often.

B vitamins in the brain-protective diet

The B-vitamin group is a family of eight vitamins, widely found in foods that are vital for health. Three in particular, vitamins B6, folate (B9) and B12, are thought to be important for a healthy brain. In addition to their role in maintaining healthy nerve cells, blood cells and genetic material, these vitamins help to control levels of a natural chemical called homocysteine, blood levels of which are higher than usual in people with dementia.

Homocysteine levels rise naturally as we age and for years it was thought that high homocysteine increased the risk of heart disease and stroke. Despite research showing that supplementing with one or more of the three B vitamins lowers homocysteine, the risk of heart disease and dementia has not always been reduced. This means we do not yet know whether high homocysteine levels are a risk factor for dementia and AD or simply a sign of the underlying disease processes that cause them. However, high homocysteine levels or low levels of B vitamins have been linked to damage to nerve cells and blood vessels, both of which are involved in the development of dementia.

Know your B vitamins
- Vitamin B6 helps us to use and store energy from food as well as helping to make hemoglobin, the red pigment in blood that carries oxygen to our cells. It also supports the immune system and is involved in producing the brain chemicals serotonin and noradrenaline (norepinephrine), which affect mood.
- Folate is important for cell division and making DNA and red blood cells.
- Vitamin B12 also makes DNA and helps keep the nervous system and blood cells healthy. It also helps prevent a type of anemia called megaloblastic anemia.

Food sources
Vitamin B6 is found in a wide range of foods, with meat, fish, poultry, liver, whole grains, potatoes, vegetables, some fruits and nuts and some fortified products all being good sources.

Folate is also found in a wide range of foods such as liver, yeast extract, beans, pulses and green leafy vegetables such as broccoli, asparagus and Brussels sprouts. Bread, cereals, pasta and other grain products are fortified with folic acid by law in the US, but not in the UK, although some cereals may be fortified. The synthetic form, folic acid, is more easily absorbed than natural folate.

Vitamin B12 is found in animal products such as meat, offal, molluscs, fish, milk, cheese and eggs (see Appendix 3 for a detailed list). The amount of vitamin B12 that we can absorb and use from these foods varies. People with reduced stomach acid or a lack of a compound called Intrinsic Factor may not be able to absorb and use the B12 from food very well.

Reduced stomach acid is relatively common in older age, but can also be due to medications such as proton-pump inhibitors designed to reduce stomach acid in people with gastro-esophageal reflux. Some diabetic medications, such as Metformin, also reduce B12 absorption. A condition called pernicious anemia results in an inability to absorb B12.

Not all foods containing B vitamins are created equal and our bodies find it easier to absorb and use the B12 and folate present in milk than the same vitamins present in meat.

What is the evidence?
There is a strong interrelationship between vitamin B6, folate and B12, although most research on dementia has focused on vitamin B12 and folate. Observational studies have found a strong correlation between high homocysteine, low B-vitamin levels and cognitive impairment/dementia, and several reviews have addressed whether this is cause or effect. Although the results are not conclusive, there is some evidence that a high homocysteine level may increase the risk of AD and dementia and that low folate and possibly low B12 levels may be risk factors.

FOLATE OR FOLIC ACID— WHAT'S THE DIFFERENCE?

Folate is the natural form of vitamin B9 found in food. Folic acid is the synthetic form of the same vitamin found in supplements and fortified foods.

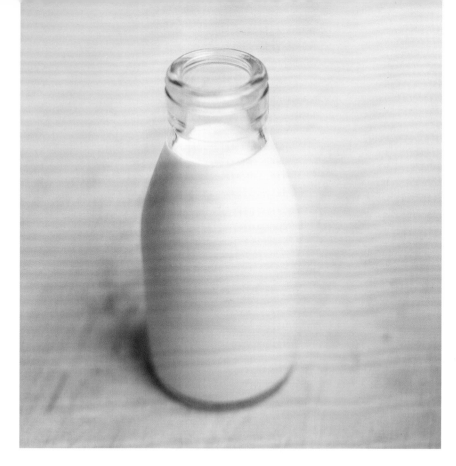

So could supplementary B vitamins improve cognition? A number of clinical trials have attempted to answer this in both people with healthy brain function and those with dementia. Most show that B-vitamin supplements reduce homocysteine levels as well as increasing levels of vitamin B. Unfortunately this is not always accompanied by an improvement in brain function.

There are many possible reasons why trial results have been inconsistent, including:

- differences in the way studies were carried out and in the dose of vitamins used
- too few study participants or not running the trial for long enough
- the use of different types of supplement and different ways of administering them (e.g. oral B12 versus B12 injections)
- not accounting for people's starting levels of vitamin B6, folate and B12
- the presence of other health problems, such as low levels of stomach acid, which reduces B12 absorption, or kidney disease, which also causes high homocysteine levels.

Some studies are more encouraging. One of the best known is a well-conducted clinical trial of 168 older people from the Oxford area in the UK published in 2010. This found that a B-vitamin supplement of folic acid, vitamin B12 and vitamin B6 reduced the rate of brain shrinkage (atrophy) in people with mild cognitive impairment (MCI). Specifically, when viewed on MRI scans, the brains of those who took B vitamins shrank 31 percent more slowly than the brains of those who took a placebo. This effect was even more marked in those who started out with the highest homocysteine level, whose brains shrank 53 percent more slowly.

A more detailed analysis of the Oxford trial by the same researchers published in 2013 found a sevenfold reduction of atrophy in areas of the brain especially vulnerable to AD in those who took B vitamins. The benefits of supplementation in this trial were confined to those who had high homocysteine levels at the outset. What this study doesn't tell us is whether B vitamins can delay the onset of dementia. But, as the brain shrinks faster in people with MCI who subsequently develop Alzheimer's disease, it could be possible.

How do they work?

There is still a lot to learn about how B vitamins may help keep the brain healthy. But what we do know is that high homocysteine levels may contribute to dementia directly, by causing nerve cells to die, and indirectly, by damaging blood vessels. So, in theory at least, lowering homocysteine levels with B vitamins could reduce dementia risk. By the same token, higher levels of B vitamins might reduce the rate of brain shrinkage, which in turn could slow cognitive decline. Some studies have also linked raised blood homocysteine levels to higher levels of Aβ proteins in the blood, although it is still unclear whether blood levels of Aβ (as opposed to the presence of Aβ in the brain) are a mark of cognitive decline.

Are we getting enough?
The average UK adult daily intake of vitamin B6 and B12 is above the UK recommended nutrient intake (RNI) of 1.2–1.4 milligrams and 1.5 micrograms a day respectively, according to the UK National Diet and Nutrition Survey (NDNS) published in 2014, which provides a picture of the food and nutrient intake of people living in the UK. The average daily intake of folate for adults is only just above the UK RNI of 200 micrograms per day, with between 1 and 3 percent of adults not getting enough. However, some studies suggest that 20 percent of people in industrialized countries are short of B12.

Recommendations
While there is currently no good evidence that taking a B-vitamin supplement will reduce dementia, supplements taken at an early stage in the disease (mild cognitive impairment) were shown in the Oxford trial to slow cognitive decline, so we recommend ensuring an adequate intake of B vitamins by the following means:

- Increase your intake of foods rich in vitamin B6 (see Appendix 3). Aim for around 1.5 milligrams a day from food and/or supplements but no more than 200 milligrams per day.
- Aim to get at least 200 micrograms (and preferably 400 micrograms) of folate a day from food and/or supplements by consuming plenty of fresh foods rich in folate (see Appendix 3), especially those like milk,

where the folate is readily available. Avoid consuming more than 1,000 micrograms a day (1 milligram a day) from fortified foods or supplements except on medical advice.
- In the US, a crystalline form of B12 (cyanocobalamin) that is easily absorbed is found in supplements and fortified foods. The US institute of Medicine (IOM) recommends that people aged over 50 should get most of their B12 in this form.
- In the UK, where only some breakfast cereals are fortified with vitamin B12, aim to eat more foods containing B12. The B12 in milk is especially easy to absorb (see Appendix 3 for other good sources).
- If you are over 50, consider taking a B-complex supplement containing a mix of all the B vitamins. Look for one that supplies around 25 micrograms a day of vitamin B12. This will provide enough to be absorbed even if you have low levels of stomach acid.

Points to note
Vitamin B6
- You should be able to get all the vitamin B6 you need from your diet. High-dose supplements (200–700 milligrams a day) can cause potentially irreversible nerve damage when taken for more than a few weeks. An "upper intake level" of 100 milligrams per day (adults) should be safe.
- As B6 supplements interact with certain medications used to treat epilepsy, TB and lung disease, seek medical advice before taking a supplement if you are affected.

Folic acid
- Consuming more than 1 milligram of folic acid a day from fortified foods or

supplements can mask symptoms of megaloblastic anemia, a type of anemia associated with vitamin B12 deficiency that can result in nerve damage.
- Modest amounts of folic acid may reduce the risk of some cancers such as colon cancer. However, there is concern that supplementing with high levels of supplemental folic acid may speed up the growth of existing tumours.

B12
- So long as you are healthy you are unlikely to experience any harm from too much B12 from food or supplements.
- Older people are more at risk of B12 deficiency because it is harder for them to absorb it.

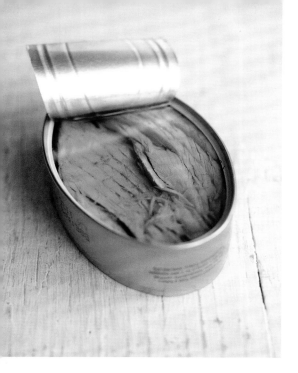

Vitamin D in the brain-protective diet

Vitamin D, which strictly speaking is not a vitamin but a hormone, has long been known to prevent bone diseases such as rickets in children and its adult equivalent, osteomalacia. It helps us to absorb calcium and works with other hormones to control the levels of calcium and phosphorous in the blood, which in turn keeps our bones, muscles and nerves healthy.

In the last few years there has been an explosion of research into vitamin D, with suggestions that it may have much wider health benefits. These include improving heart health and immune function and helping to protect against certain cancers and dementia. Research into how vitamin D works in the brain is growing. It is thought to have a role in controlling certain genes and scientists also suggest that it may reduce inflammation and clear Aβ protein from the brain, although this still has to be proved.

Food sources

Most vitamin D does not come from food but from the action of UVB in sunlight on a cholesterol compound in the skin (see figure opposite). Foods that contain vitamin D include oily fish, liver, eggs and sun-dried shiitake mushrooms or ordinary button mushrooms exposed to sunlight or artificial UV light.

The vitamin D in food can be either D3 (cholecalciferol) or D2 (ergocaciferol). Both are used in food supplements and fortified foods, although it appears that vitamin D2 is less biologically active. Most industrialized countries fortify some foods with vitamin D, including breakfast cereals and margarines. Milk is fortified with vitamin D2 in the US but not the UK.

What is the evidence?

The risk of dementia increases significantly with age and low levels of vitamin D are common in older people. Numerous studies have compared the vitamin D levels of people with dementia with those without and there has also been extensive research comparing how people perform in tests of mental function with their vitamin D level. Research includes:

- a large analysis of seven studies published in 2012 that suggested that vitamin D deficiency more than doubled the risk of cognitive impairment
- another analysis of 37 studies, which concluded that lower vitamin D levels were associated with poorer cognitive function as well as with a higher risk of developing AD
- a 2013 review of 18 out of 25 studies, which showed that lower levels of vitamin D were associated with poorer cognitive function; people with lower vitamin D levels at the start of a study were also at a higher risk of cognitive decline four to seven years later
- a 2013 Dutch study of 127 older people, which found that those with lower levels of vitamin D in their blood performed worse on tests involving executive function and processing speed, suggesting that vitamin D may be involved in specific cognitive areas
- a large, long-term study of 10,186 Danes published in 2013, noting an increased risk of developing AD as blood levels of vitamin D decreased over a 30-year period.

DID YOU KNOW?

Placing any variety of mushrooms in the sun for around 30 minutes will result in the production of around 10 micrograms (400 IU) of vitamin D2 per 80 grams (3 ounces), according to US vitamin-D researcher Dr. Michael Hollick.

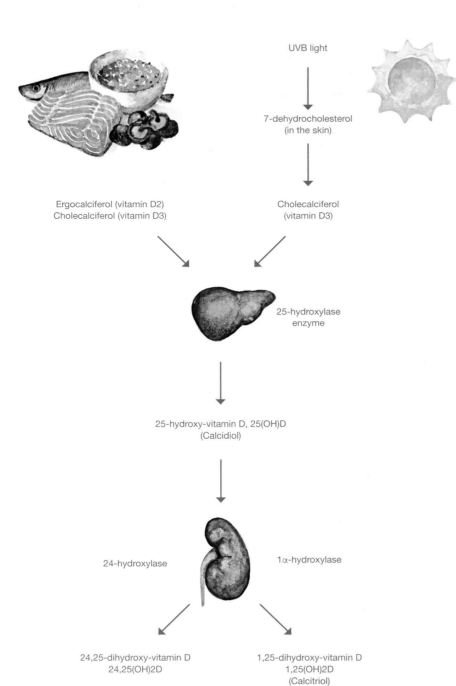

UVB light

7-dehydrocholesterol
(in the skin)

Ergocalciferol (vitamin D2)
Cholecalciferol (vitamin D3)

Cholecalciferol
(vitamin D3)

25-hydroxylase
enzyme

25-hydroxy-vitamin D, 25(OH)D
(Calcidiol)

24-hydroxylase

1α-hydroxylase

24,25-dihydroxy-vitamin D
24,25(OH)2D

1,25-dihydroxy-vitamin D
1,25(OH)2D
(Calcitriol)

**This illustration shows
how the inactive vitamin
D forms, vitamin D2
(ergocalciferol) and vitamin
D3 (cholecalciferol), are
converted into a form of
vitamin D known as 25(OH)
D (calcidiol) in the liver.
From here it circulates in
the blood to the kidneys and
other tissues, including the
brain, where it is converted
to the active form of vitamin
D, known as 1,25(OH)2D or
calcitriol.**

As with other nutrients, although observational studies suggest a strong link between vitamin D and dementia, they do not prove that vitamin D deficiency causes dementia nor that vitamin D supplementation prevents it. To date, there have been no high-quality clinical trials investigating the effect of vitamin D supplementation alone on the development of dementia.

One trial that set out to test whether vitamin D and calcium supplementation could protect against cognitive decline compared the effects of taking 1,000 milligrams of calcium plus 400 IU of vitamin D daily with taking a placebo on the risk of cognitive impairment or dementia in 4,143 women aged 64 or over. There was no reduction in dementia or signs of cognitive impairment in those who took the supplement after approximately seven years. Potential reasons for this disappointing result include the following:

- the design of the trial meant that any effects lower than a reduction in risk of one-third would not have been detected
- participants were relatively young and their cognitive function relatively high at the start of the trial (high cognition is protective against dementia)
- vitamin D levels were only measured in 150 people in the supplemented group at the start and not again at the end, so it is not known whether the supplements had any effect on vitamin D status.

Future trials looking at vitamin D supplementation will have to take into account the amount of sunlight received by participants as well as the fact that the current method of using 25(OH)D

KNOW YOUR VITAMIN D LEVEL

The active form of vitamin D [1,25(OH)2D] is only present in the bloodstream for a few hours, so levels of the inactive form, 25(OH)D, in blood are used to determine vitamin D level.

There is still debate over the ideal level of vitamin D but the following blood levels of 25(OH)D are widely accepted:
- deficient—below 25 nanomoles per liter (nmol/L)
- insufficient—between 25–50 nmol/L
- desirable—75 nmol/L or above.

Ask your doctor for a blood test to check your vitamin D level if you think you might be at risk of deficiency.

as a measure of vitamin D status only shows vitamin D levels over the previous few weeks, so cannot estimate the potential effects of long-term vitamin D deficiency.

How does it work?
Vitamin D acts through special receptors found in several different tissues and controls the action of more than 200 genes, directly or indirectly, through these receptors. More specifically, these receptors are found in nerve cells in the part of the brain critical for cognition and it is thought that their number reduces as we age. We now know that brain cells have the ability to produce the enzyme needed to convert 25(OH)D to the active form.

Scientists are still unsure exactly how vitamin D affects cognition. However, it has an important role in nerve cell growth and survival. It also has the ability to affect levels of certain brain chemicals, such as acetylcholine, a messenger chemical found in the brain that is important for memory. These functions

all add up to the belief that vitamin D is an important nutrient when it comes to maintaining brain health and suggest viable biological mechanisms through which it may provide protection.

Are we getting enough?
Vitamin D insufficiency and deficiency are common worldwide in those with limited exposure to sunlight. At-risk groups include young children, pregnant women, older people, dark-skinned people, people who wear enveloping clothing and those living in northern countries.

As food is a poor source of vitamin D, we rely on exposing our skin to sunlight to ensure we get enough. Unfortunately many parts of the world are on too low a latitude to ensure that this happens all year round. In the UK, for example, which lies between 50° and 57° latitude, the sun is too low in the sky between October and the end of March. The result? Many Britons have sub-optimal levels or are vitamin-D deficient during winter and spring. During the rest of the year more than half the effective UV radiation occurs between 11am and 3pm. Other factors such as cloud cover and pollution can also reduce exposure. A simple rule of thumb is that you only make vitamin D in the skin when your shadow is shorter than your height.

The recommended daily allowance (RDA) set by the Institute of Medicine (IOM) in the US is 15 micrograms (600 IU) a day for adults up to the age of 70 and 20 micrograms (800 IU) a day for those over 70. The UK currently has no figure for adults below the age of 65 (unless pregnant). The Scientific Advisory Committee on Nutrition (SACN) is currently looking at this and is expected to recommend a daily intake level for adults in the near future, so watch this space.

Recommendations

It is difficult to make general recommendations as so many different factors are involved and there is no firm agreement among scientists as to the ideal level of vitamin D. However, after taking into account recommendations from other bodies* we suggest the following:

- Include plenty of vitamin-D rich foods in your diet (see Appendix 3).
- Expose forearms and partially covered legs (around 18 percent of the body) to the sun without sunscreen for approximately 15 minutes a day between 10am and 3pm, but avoid excessive sun exposure due to the increased risk of skin cancer.
- If you are unable to get enough sun exposure, or are in an at-risk group, consider taking a vitamin D supplement of up to 25 micrograms (1,000 IU) per day. This is close to the USA recommendation of 20 micrograms (800 IU) per day for those aged 71 or over and well below the US Institute of Medicine's safe upper limit of 100 micrograms (4,000 IU) per day.
- Overt vitamin D deficiency should be corrected under the guidance of a medical practitioner and individuals who are abnormally sensitive to vitamin D (for example people with granulomatous disorders) should always seek medical advice.

Note: One microgram of dietary vitamin D = 40 international units (IU).
For blood levels, 2.5 nmol/L of 25(OH)D = 1 ng/ml.

* The International Osteoporosis Foundation, the Endocrine Society and a Polish multidisciplinary group that recently published recommendations for Central Europeans. These are not specific to dementia.

Points to note

- You can't get too much vitamin D from sunlight. Once your skin has made enough (usually when it goes slightly red), production is switched off. However, remember that excessive exposure to sunlight increases the risk of skin cancer, so avoid too much sun exposure.
- Large intakes of vitamin D from supplements can lead to high levels of calcium in the blood (hypercalcaemia), which in turn can lead to kidney failure and cardiac arrest.
- The EU Scientific Committee on Food and the US Institute of Medicine recommend an "upper intake level" of 100 micrograms (4,000 IU) a day for adults. The UK Expert Group on Vitamins and Minerals suggests that, taken regularly over a long period, a supplement of 25 micrograms (1,000 IU) a day is unlikely to cause harm.

ARE YOU AT RISK?

You may be at risk of vitamin D deficiency if you:
- live in a country above or below 50° latitude
- don't spend much time outdoors
- have dark skin
- are over the age of 65—elderly skin makes less vitamin D
- use sunscreen as soon as you go in the sun
- wear clothing that leaves very little skin exposed
- are obese or suffer from a malabsorption syndrome, such as Crohn's disease

Fats and fish for brain-protection

We all need some fat in our diet to give us energy, help us absorb the fat-soluble vitamins A, D, E and K and some plant chemicals, and enable our cell membranes, including those in the brain, to function properly. Certain fats can help protect the brain. However, too much fat, or too much of certain kinds of fats, may increase the risk of health problems, including cognitive decline and dementia.

Omega-3s and brain health

One of the most important things you can do to help keep your brain healthy is to eat fish—and the oilier, the better. Oily fish such as salmon, herring, mackerel, sardines and tuna contain the two special long-chain marine omega-3s, eicosapentanoic acid (EPA) and docosahexanoic acid (DHA), that are essential throughout life for a healthy brain. DHA appears especially important for a sharp brain as we age.

The brain is a fatty organ and its cells, and the connections between them, are rich in DHA. But as we get older, DHA levels dwindle. People with cognitive impairment and often with Alzheimer's disease have lower DHA levels too, although whether this is a cause or an effect of the disease process is not known. Marine omega-3s also play a key role in heart health—and what is good for the heart is good for the brain. Numerous studies have investigated the effects of fish or long-chain marine omega-3s on brain function and, on the whole, they appear to be protective. What

KNOW YOUR FATTY ACIDS

Fatty acids, the building blocks of fat, come in several forms.

Saturated fatty acids (SFA), found mainly in red and processed meats, butter, cream, whole milk, cheese, cakes, pastries and cookies, are hard at room temperature. In some studies a high intake has been linked to an increased risk of cognitive decline and dementia.

Unsaturated fatty acids, found in fish, vegetables, nuts, seeds and their oils, are liquid at room temperature. Studies link certain unsaturated fatty acids with a lower risk of cognitive decline and dementia. Key ones include:

1. **Polyunsaturated fatty acids (PUFA)**, of which there are two important kinds—omega-6 fatty acids and omega-3 fatty acids. Omega-6s are found in nuts, seeds and grains, vegetable oils such as corn oil, soybean oil, sunflower oil and spreads made from these. Omega-3s may be "long-chain marine omega-3s" from fish and seafood, or "medium-chain plant omega-3s" from flaxseed, canola, walnuts and their oils, and green leafy vegetables.

2. **Monounsaturated fatty acids (MUFA)**, found in foods such as olives and avocados and in oils such as olive oil or canola oil, often sold in supermarkets simply as "vegetable oil." They include the omega-9 fatty acid oleic acid, found in olive oil, and have been linked with a lower risk of cognitive decline, especially as part of the Mediterranean diet.

Trans-fats
Trans-fats also come in two forms:
1. **Industrial trans-fats** found in processed foods—such as spreads, bought cookies, cakes, pastries, prepared food and takeouts—are vegetable oils, which have been processed (hydrogenated) to stop them going rancid and preserve shelf life. Studies show that industrial trans-fats (look for labels reading "hydrogenated" or "partially hydrogenated") are especially harmful to the heart, and although this is less widely researched, to brain health.

2. **Natural trans-fats** from certain animals, such as sheep and cows, are found in meat and in small amounts in dairy products, such as butter. The few studies carried out on these suggest that they may have similar effects if consumed in the same high amounts as industrial trans-fats. On a daily basis, however, we usually only consume small amounts.

THE LONG AND THE SHORT OF IT

Fatty acids can be short, medium, long or very long-chain. When it comes to brain health the long-chain marine omega-3s, EPA and DHA from fish and seafood, seem to be the ones that count rather than the shorter-chain plant omega-3, alpha-linolenic acid (ALA), found in flaxseed, canola, walnuts and their oils. ALA is used to make EPA and DHA. However, although children can convert ALA to EPA and DHA, as adults we lose this ability. EPA and DHA come pre-formed in fish and seafood, which is why fish is so important for a healthy brain.

is still not clear is whether long-chain marine omega-3s—specifically DHA—are the secret to the brain-protective benefits observed, or whether other factors or nutrients may be responsible. Fish is also a source of protein, taurine (the "free" amino acid), vitamin D, B vitamins, selenium, zinc and iodine, all of which may help protect against cognitive decline.

Food sources

Oily fish such as herring, mackerel, trout, tuna (fresh or frozen, not canned), sprats, salmon, sardines, swordfish, marlin, kippers, pilchards and whitebait are the best sources of long-chain marine omega-3s. White fish—cod, haddock, plaice, pollack, coley, Dover sole, dab, flounder, red mullet and gurnard—and shellfish such as shrimp and crab also contain some. Omega-3-enriched eggs, spreads and breads, and some brands of milk and

yogurt are sources of omega-3s if you are vegetarian or don't eat fish. However, as these are the shorter-chain plant omega-3s, they may not protect the brain.

What is the evidence?

Rates of Alzheimer's disease are lower in places such as Japan, where people traditionally eat more fish than in Europe and the USA. Older Japanese men living in America, for example, are two and a half times more likely to develop AD than their peers living in Japan. Interestingly, rates of AD have started to creep up in Japan—from around 1 percent in 1985 to around 7 percent in 2008. The population of Japan is aging like that of other countries, which could be one reason for this increase. However, the rise also parallels a change to a more Westernized diet containing less fish and more meat and animal fat.

Observational studies, carried out in countries as far apart as France, the Netherlands, Scandinavia and the US, strongly suggest that regularly eating fish—especially those long-chain omega-3-rich oily fish—may slow cognitive decline and/or reduce the risk of dementia or AD. However, not all studies are favorable and in some that are, the benefits only apply to people who do not carry the ApoE ε4 gene variant, which is the most important genetic risk factor for AD. One clue as to the reason for this is that, in mice at least, ApoE ε4 appears to block uptake of DHA by the brain.

Another reason for unclear results may be that other factors rather than fish intake or DHA account for the findings. A 2005 French study, for example, found that people who ate fish more often tended to be more highly educated, which can

make the brain more resilient to dementia. They were also more likely to eat a healthy diet, rich in pulses, fruit and vegetables, to drink alcohol, report better health and be less depressed—all factors that have been linked with a lower risk of dementia.

How often should you eat fish?

Studies suggest that for optimum benefit, fish needs to go on the menu at least once a week.

- A US study that looked at the diets of people living in south Chicago found that those who ate fish at least once a week had a 10 percent slower rate of cognitive decline than those who ate fish rarely or never.
- A study in the French cities of Bordeaux, Montpellier and Dijon showed that eating fish on a weekly basis was linked with a 40 percent lower risk of dementia and a 35 percent lower risk of AD—but only in people without the ε4 variant of the ApoE gene.
- In the US Framingham Study, a large study originally set up to track risk factors for heart disease, people who ate fish on average three times a week had higher blood levels of DHA together with a 39 percent lower risk of AD and a 47 percent lower risk of dementia.

Does the type of fish matter?

Studies suggest that the type of fish and how it is cooked may be important. Dark-fleshed fin fish such as dark tuna, herring, mackerel and sardines are a good choice and baking or grilling rather than frying is the best way to reap their benefits. Fish burgers, fish fingers and other manufactured fish products are unlikely to be beneficial, according to research.

How does it work?

DHA may help to:

- quell brain inflammation
- increase production of protective anti-inflammatory chemicals
- increase the fluidity of cell membranes
- maintain connections between brain cells (synapses) and help prevent their loss
- stop the loss of brain cells caused by overzealous programmed cell death (apoptosis)
- prevent formation of protein "plaques and tangles"
- improve the brain's ability to respond to insulin
- improve atherosclerosis (hardened and narrowed arteries), blood pressure and elasticity of the blood vessels, which are linked to a higher risk of vascular dementia and AD
- increase the formation of new nerve cells (neurogenesis)
- prevent the silent lesions (subclinical infarcts) that increase the risk of cognitive decline and dementia
- preserve the brain's white matter, damage to which is linked to cognitive impairment.

Are we getting enough?

The amount of fish eaten around the world varies enormously, with Asian countries leading the way and Western countries tending to lag behind.

- In the UK, fish intake is just 63 grams (2¼ ounces) a week of white, coated or fried fish, 140 grams (5 ounces) a week of other white fish, shellfish, fish dishes and canned tuna and just 91 grams (3¼ ounces) a week of the oily fish thought to benefit the brain most.
- In the US, consumption is 91 grams/ 3¼ ounces (prepared weight) of fish and shellfish a week.
- In both countries, intake falls short of the amounts recommended for health. In the UK this is two portions of fish (140 grams/5 ounces per portion cooked weight) a week, one of which should be oily; and in the US it is 226–340 grams (8–12 ounces) a week, an amount providing approximately 250 milligrams of long-chain omega-3 fatty acids a day.

SAFETY AND SUSTAINABILITY

Sadly, the sea and rivers can contain potentially harmful mercury and other pollutants, which can accumulate in fish such as shark, swordfish and marlin. This is why experts recommend limiting fish consumption to no more than four portions of oily fish a week. There is also the problem of overfishing. You can help ease strain on world fish stocks by choosing sustainable fish and seafood. Visit www.fishonline.org.

Recommendations

These studies have produced mixed results, but fish is, generally speaking, extremely healthy and may help to keep the brain sharp if you eat it regularly, especially in middle age.

- Aim for at least two portions of fish a week and make at least one of these oily.
- An average portion is 140 grams (5 ounces) but can range from around 100 to 200 grams (3½–7 ounces).
- For optimum benefit it may be worth putting a second, third or even fourth portion of fish on the menu each week—no more than this, though, to avoid the risks of pollution.
- Wild oily fish are generally richer in omega-3s than farmed varieties, as the omega-3 content of farmed fish depends on the amount of marine oil in their feed.
- The best cooking methods are baking or grilling. Avoid frying, which may reduce or negate the benefits of fish oils.
- Plant-based omega-3s from foods such as flaxseed, walnuts and their oils, as well as canola oil and green leafy vegetables, don't benefit the brain directly but can help lower cholesterol levels, which can indirectly help keep your brain healthy.

TO SUPPLEMENT OR NOT?

Most experts agree that eating fish is the best way to benefit from the fats and other potentially brain-friendly nutrients they contain. Results of clinical trials that have attempted to discover whether fish-oil supplements may improve brain function, in people with healthy brains or those with mild cognitive impairment or AD, have been inconsistent; but by and large they show no clear benefit.

A 2012 review from the Cochrane Collaboration, an organization that assesses medical research to reach evidence-based conclusions, concluded that neither DHA nor fish oils, when taken as supplements, protected against cognitive decline or dementia in the over-60s with healthy brain function, although longer studies might be needed to detect an effect. Several studies are ongoing and may in time help to clarify who, if anyone, might benefit from taking a supplement, the optimum dose and the stage in life at which it may be beneficial.

Point to note
Check food packs carefully. Some products, such as canola oil and spreads (soft margarines), labeled as being a source of omega-3s, may in fact contain the less brain-protective medium-chain plant omega-3, ALA.

Omega-6s and brain health

Like omega-3s, the other main family of polyunsaturated fatty acids, omega-6s, are vital for health but scientists are still arguing about how much we need. Early research focused on the cholesterol-lowering, heart-protective benefits of omega-6s. More recently, research has found that omega-6s are also vital for brain growth and cognitive development, as well as helping to lower

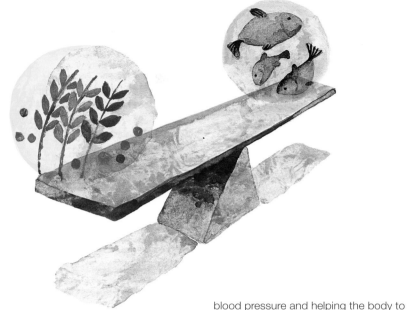

Omega-6s one end and Omega-3s the other

blood pressure and helping the body to deal with insulin, all of which may make them useful in helping prevent dementia. However, studies suggest that too many omega-6s or too high a ratio to omega-3s could be detrimental.

Food sources
Omega-6s are found in nuts, seeds and oils, such as corn oil, safflower oil, sunflower oil, soy oil, peanut oil, spreads and many processed foods.

What is the evidence?
In one of the earliest studies looking at the potential links between fat intake and dementia, carried out in Zutphen, a small city in the eastern Netherlands, a high intake of the omega-6 fatty acid linoleic acid was linked to a higher risk of cognitive impairment in a group of older men aged from 69 to 89 years. More recently a Greek study, which examined the brain health of older people living in and around Athens, also found that those who consumed a higher intake

A QUESTION OF BALANCE?

Our hunter-gatherer ancestors are thought to have consumed a ratio of 1:1 or 2:1 omega-6s to omega-3s. These days we consume them in a ratio more like 15:1 or even 25:1. In other words we are consuming 15 to 25 times as many omega-6s as omega-3s, far more than our distant forebears. And this, according to a German review published in 2014, could be detrimental to the brain. The authors concluded that a low omega-6 to omega-3 ratio could help preserve cognitive function and play a part in preventing dementia.

Animal studies show that reducing the amount of dietary omega-6s boosts metabolism of the brain-healthy

omega-3s and increases the concentration of anti-inflammatory chemicals in the brain. It is not known if this applies to humans, but it is interesting that the Mediterranean diet, which, according to many health professionals is healthier for the body and brain, has a more balanced ratio of these two fatty-acid families.

Other scientists, however, argue that lumping all omega-3s and omega-6s together is not useful and that, rather than focusing on ratios, we should be trying to establish which particular fatty acids have what effects and how much of them we need.

of omega-6s, mainly linoleic acid from seed oils, had poorer cognitive function. Meanwhile, in a well-known French study looking at the health of older people in Montpellier, Bordeaux and Dijon, regular consumption of omega-6 rich oils, not counterbalanced by consumption of omega-3 rich oils or fish, was linked to a doubling of the risk of dementia in people without the ApoE ε4 gene variant—in other words, in people with no increased risk of AD from their genes. In another French study, high levels of omega-6s were consistently linked with a higher risk of cognitive decline.

Recommendations

The jury is still out on the optimum amount of omega-6s for a healthy brain, but for heart health, which has a known impact on the brain, many health officials recommend that they should provide around 4 percent of calories a day— around 8–10 grams (¼ ounce) a day. The American Heart Association, on the other hand, recommends that omega-6s make up to around 10 percent of calories a day.

We recommend the following:

- Limit consumption of soft margarines and processed foods containing omega-6s, such as crisps and other savory snacks, crackers and fast foods.
- Cook as much food as you can yourself, using healthier oils such as canola oil or olive oil.
- Nuts contain omega-6s. However, they also contain other beneficial nutrients, such as medium-chain omega-3s, MUFAs, vitamin E, a variety of minerals and other heart- and potentially brain-friendly nutrients. Walnuts, for example, helped improve memory and learning in one study in rats. Use them in stir-fries, pesto and salads. But don't go overboard as they are high in calories.

MUFAs and the brain

Much studied for their benefits for heart health, monounsaturated fatty acids (MUFAs), found in olive oil, are especially resistant to the oxidation thought to play such an important role in the development of both heart disease and dementia. MUFAs are also key ingredients of the Mediterranean diet and may be one of the reasons it is so healthy for the body and brain.

Food sources

Olive oil contains a high percentage— around 70 to 80 percent—of MUFAs, mainly in the form of an omega-9 fatty acid, oleic acid, together with a small percentage (around 8–10 percent) of polyunsaturated fatty acids (PUFAs). MUFAs are also found in olives, avocados, some nuts and canola oil.

OLIVE OIL—MORE THAN MUFAS

Olive oil is also a rich source of other nutrients and plant compounds that could have brain-protective properties. These include vitamin E and a variety of polyphenols (see page 18). One polyphenol, oleocanthal, helped clear Aβ protein from the brain in a 2013 study. This finding could be part of the bigger picture of the potential brain-enhancing properties of olive oil.

What is the evidence?

MUFAs have been linked with sharper brain function in several research projects. One study, published in 1999, which examined the diets of a group of 65- to 84-year-olds in northern, central and southern Italy, found that those with a high intake of MUFAs had a lower risk of cognitive decline, a finding confirmed in 2006 after researchers had followed up the participants for eight and a half years.

Ten years later a French study, looking specifically at olive-oil intake in healthy older inhabitants of Dijon, Montpellier and Bordeaux, found that those most liberal with the olive oil—meaning that they used it in both cooking and dressings—had a 17 percent lower risk of a decline in visual memory than those who used none.

These findings are echoed in other studies. However, as with so much dietary research, it is uncertain whether the effects observed are due to MUFAs, whether a high MUFA intake is a marker of a healthy eating pattern, or whether the apparent benefits are in fact due to other components of MUFA-rich foods.

How do they work?

MUFAs are known for their ability to help maintain a healthy cholesterol profile, help blood clot normally and enhance insulin control, all of which may benefit the brain. MUFAs can also help to maintain the health of the thin layer of cells that lines the blood vessels (endothelium), quell oxidative stress and keep a lid on inflammation.

As for direct effects on the brain, MUFAs may help maintain the structure of brain-cell membranes and help keep the connections between brain cells healthy so they are better able to communicate. Oleic acid, especially, may have more specific benefits. In mice, for example, a low-fat, high-oleic-acid diet was found to help prevent the formation of Aβ plaques.

Recommendations

Most experts agree that more studies are needed but, in light of their known heart benefits, it is worth replacing some of the saturated and trans-fats in your diet with olive oil and other MUFA-rich foods. In Mediterranean countries, olive oil consumption typically amounts to 46 grams (just over four tablespoons) a day, an amount you should be able to achieve without too much effort. But even smaller amounts could have benefits.

- Try dipping bread in olive oil, use canola oil for frying or sautéing and use olive oil in sauces, toppings and dressings.
- Unlike omega-6 vegetable oils, such as corn, sunflower, safflower or soy oil, olive oil is less likely to go rancid and keeps well in the cupboard.
- Extra-virgin olive oil may be especially healthy used cold in dressings and toppings because it contains several ingredients from olive leaves and skin not found in oils manufactured from seeds or grains.
- Remember, like all fats, MUFAs are high in calories, so use them instead of other less healthy fats, such as saturated and trans-fats—but don't go overboard.

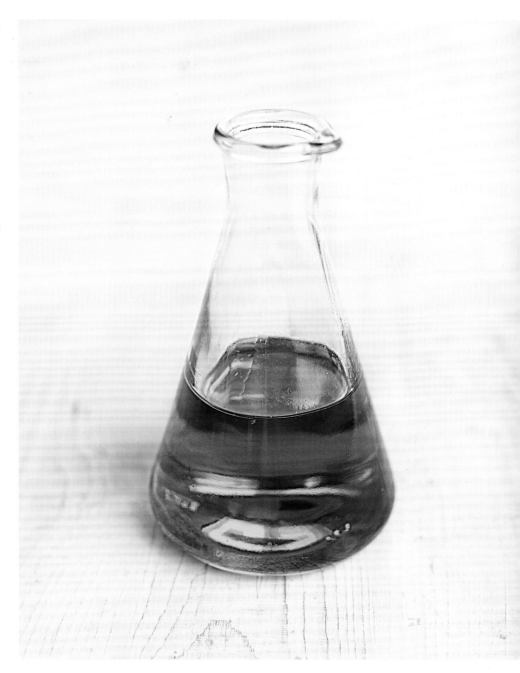

Saturated and trans-fats and the brain

Despite the beneficial effect of some fats on the risk of cognitive decline and dementia, other fats are less beneficial. The chief culprits are saturated fats, found in meat, cheese, butter, cakes, pastries and baked goods, and manufactured trans-fats, found in processed foods.

What is the evidence?
Many studies suggest that a diet high in saturated and trans-fats increases the risk of cognitive decline and dementia. An influential project, which is studying the role of diet and other environmental factors on the risk of dementia in older residents of Chicago, found that healthy older people who consumed the most saturated fats had more than double the risk of Alzheimer's disease of those who consumed the least. A high trans-fat intake was also associated with a higher risk of cognitive problems.

Another long-running project, which started in Finland in the 1970s, also found that people with a high saturated fat intake (more than 21.5g a day) during middle age had double the risk of mild cognitive impairment later in life. The risk was especially marked among those with the ApoE ε4 gene variant. This is one of a growing number of studies suggesting that a healthy diet and lifestyle in middle age may help protect against dementia.

Saturated and trans-fats may be especially harmful if you have other risk factors for dementia. In a long-running US study of factors influencing women's health, for example, older women with type-2 diabetes whose diets were high in saturated and trans-fats experienced the worst cognitive decline.

It is less clear if a high fat intake generally contributes to a higher dementia risk. However, the overall balance of different nutrients or fats may be important. In the Finnish study already outlined, a higher ratio of polyunsaturated fats to saturated fats, as part of an overall healthy diet during middle age, was linked to better mental function in later life.

Similarly, a small US clinical trial found that a high-fat (45 percent), high-saturated fat (25 percent), high-glycaemic index (GI) diet increased a number of chemical "markers" suggestive of Alzheimer's disease in the fluid surrounding the spinal cord. A low-fat (25 percent), low-saturated fat (less than 7 percent), low-GI diet, on the other hand, reduced them.

How may saturated and trans-fats be harmful?
At nine calories per gram, fat is the most calorific of the three major nutrients (the other two being protein and carbohydrates). As such, any kind of fat can contribute to overweight, obesity, insulin resistance and type-2 diabetes, all of which are linked to a greater risk of cognitive decline and dementia. But that is not the whole story.

Saturated and trans-fats can make brain cell membranes less fluid, hampering their ability to communicate. They can also lead to an unhealthy cholesterol profile (high levels of "bad" LDL

THE CHOLESTEROL CONUNDRUM

High cholesterol in middle age increases the risk of dementia in some studies. High cholesterol contributes to the atherosclerosis (furring and narrowing of the arteries) that increases the risk of vascular dementia and AD. It may also accelerate the formation of Aβ protein. On the other hand, high cholesterol in later life is linked with a lower risk of dementia. It is not yet clear what this may mean. However, it is certainly worth making an effort to keep cholesterol down during middle age.

cholesterol and low levels of "good" HDL cholesterol), which may be linked to an increased risk of cognitive problems. Finally, saturated and trans-fats may trigger inflammatory chemicals and increase cell death or apoptosis, which is known to be a major factor in the loss of brain cells in AD.

Recommendations
Fat remains a controversial topic constantly under debate. However, most nutrition experts still believe that for overall health—including a healthy brain—a low intake of saturated and trans-fats, together with a low intake of omega-6s, a moderate intake of monounsaturated fats (see page 32) and a moderate to high intake of long-chain omega-3s is optimal. In the absence of clear conclusions from studies, we recommend the following:
- Keep saturated fats to a minimum by choosing lower-fat cuts of meat, and cutting off visible fat.

- Watch cooking methods—grill, bake, steam or stir-fry rather than frying.
- Keep trans-fat consumption to a minimum by limiting processed foods and takeouts.
- Avoid spreads labeled hydrogenated or partially hydrogenated and choose those made from monounsaturated oils such as olive oil. Better still, use olive oil or walnut oil for dipping.

SUGGESTED INTAKE OF TOTAL, SATURATED AND TRANS-FAT

Total fat	No more than 30 percent of total calories a day—around 95g (men) and 70g (women)
Saturated fat	No more than 11 percent of total calories a day—no more than 30g (men) and 20g (women)
Trans-fat	No more than 1 or 2 percent of total calories a day—i.e. no more than 2.5 or 5g

SOURCES OF SATURATED FATS AND TRANS-FATS

Saturated fats	**Trans-fats (check ingredient lists for hydrogenated fats or hydrogenated vegetable oils)**
Fatty cuts of meat	Fried foods and takeouts
Processed and cured meat products e.g. bacon, sausages, hot dogs, salami, ham, hamburgers, prosciutto and other cured raw meats, meat pies	Dairy ice cream
Full-fat milk, evaporated milk, condensed milk	Garlic and herb baguettes
Full-fat yogurt e.g. Greek yogurt	Pastries and pies e.g. bought quiche Lorraine
Creamy desserts e.g. rice pudding, pannacotta, cheesecake	Cookies and cakes
Butter, ghee, lard	Spreadable butter
Coconut and palm oils	Pizza (bought or takeout)
Cheese, especially full-fat hard and cream cheeses	
Cream, soured cream, ice cream	
Some savory snacks	
Chocolate	
Cookies, cakes, pastries	

Dietary patterns and the brain-protective diet

By now you are aware of the many nutrients and foods that may help protect you against dementia. But while this information is useful to researchers, in our everyday lives we don't sit down to a plate of vitamin E with a side of folate and an omega-3 sauce. We eat whole foods as part of complete meals and these, together with drinks and snacks, form our overall way of eating or, as nutritional researchers call it, our dietary pattern.

Many experts now argue that "food synergy" (page 8) is likely to be more important than the effects of any single nutrient and that a combination of dietary factors is likely to have the greatest effect on long-term health. This might explain why the results of some studies we have looked at have been unexpected or disappointing and why supplements don't always seem to be beneficial.

An increasing number of studies have examined the beneficial effects of different dietary patterns on the risk of diseases such as heart disease, type-2 diabetes and, in the past few years, dementia. On the whole, these appear to show stronger links than studies of single nutrients. One of the most studied has been the Mediterranean diet, although recently other dietary patterns, such as the Japanese diet, have come under the spotlight.

Mediterranean Diet Pyramid

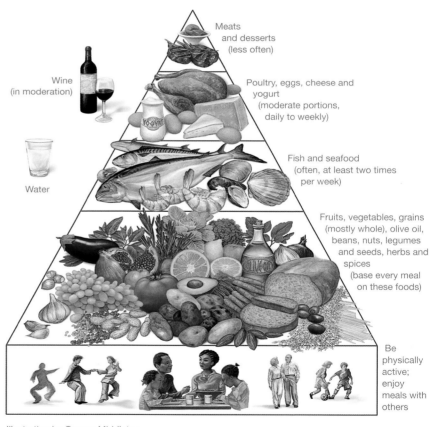

Wine (in moderation)

Water

Meats and desserts (less often)

Poultry, eggs, cheese and yogurt (moderate portions, daily to weekly)

Fish and seafood (often, at least two times per week)

Fruits, vegetables, grains (mostly whole), olive oil, beans, nuts, legumes and seeds, herbs and spices (base every meal on these foods)

Be physically active; enjoy meals with others

Illustration by George Middleton
© 2009 Oldways Preservation and Exchange Trust • www.oldwayspt.org

Consume foods at the bottom of the pyramid freely. Eat those toward the top occasionally or in small amounts.

What is the Mediterranean diet?

The Mediterranean diet is a way of eating based on foods traditionally consumed in areas that border the Mediterranean Sea, such as Crete, other parts of Greece and southern Italy. Key ingredients, usually consumed as close as possible to their natural state, are olive oil, nuts, oily fish, some poultry, a little meat, plenty of fruit, vegetables, pulses and whole grains plus a moderate amount of red wine consumed during meals. The pyramid opposite shows how they fit in to an overall eating pattern.

What is the evidence?

Numerous studies have looked at how eating the Mediterranean way may help protect against dementia.

- A 2010 analysis of 18 studies found a 13 percent reduction in the risk for neurodegenerative diseases, together with a 10 percent reduction in the risk for heart disease. The researchers concluded that, followed over a long period, a Mediterranean diet provided "significant and consistent protection against major, chronic, degenerative diseases."
- A study that analysed the results of 11 clinical trials with a total of over 50,000 participants, looking at the effect of following a Mediterranean diet on the prevention of cardiovascular disease, a key risk factor for dementia, concluded that this type of diet was very likely to help keep the heart and blood vessels healthy.
- A large analysis of 22 observational studies, published in 2013, found that sticking closely to a Mediterranean way of eating reduced the risk of stroke, another significant risk factor for dementia, by almost 30 percent, and the risk of cognitive impairment by about 40 percent.

Few clinical trials have studied the effects of a Mediterranean diet on brain function specifically. However, one that looked at the effects of an "enhanced" Mediterranean diet (with either added olive oil or extra nuts) over a period of six years found that it had beneficial effects on brain function compared to a low-fat diet.

Conflicting conclusions

Not all studies have found a positive link between a Mediterranean diet and health. This may be because people who make healthy dietary choices are more likely to have a healthy lifestyle, which can confuse results. It could also be that people whose brain function is beginning to falter may find it harder to stick to a healthy diet.

In 2013, a Scottish study initially found a link between a Mediterranean dietary pattern and better cognitive performance in old age. The association was lost, however, when they factored in the intelligence of participants. It was suggested that more intelligent people make healthier choices and so are likely to have better brain function as they get older.

A 2012 Australian study, which examined the diets of 1,500 people over four years, found that a Mediterranean-style diet provided no protection against MCI or dementia, but cooking methods (grilled fish and vegetables were more beneficial than deep-fried fish and fries) and perhaps the levels of processed versus freshly prepared foods could have skewed the results.

Other dietary patterns

The Mediterranean way of eating isn't the only one to have benefits for brain health.

- A 2013 study in Japan followed over 1,000 people for 15 years and found a reduced risk of dementia linked to a high intake of soybeans and soy products, vegetables, seaweed, milk and dairy products and a low intake of rice.
- In a multi-ethnic New York community, researchers found an average reduction of AD risk of over 35 percent in people with higher intakes of salad dressing, nuts, fish, tomatoes, poultry, cruciferous vegetables such as cabbage, broccoli and Brussels sprouts, fruit and green leafy vegetables and low intakes of high-fat dairy, red meat, offal and butter.
- In recent reviews of the evidence, a set of recommendations aimed at reducing high blood pressure known as the DASH (Dietary Approaches to Stop Hypertension) diet and a pattern of eating called the US Healthy Eating Index, 2005, has also been linked to a lower risk of dementia and AD.

Adapting your diet

We live in a global economy where foods from all over the world are readily available. However, adopting eating and cooking styles from other parts of the world is not always easy. The good news is that it is possible to adapt your own food likes and dislikes to include the beneficial components of a healthy dietary pattern wherever you live.

In compiling our recipe collection, we have identified common features of apparently beneficial dietary patterns to produce a range of dishes that we hope will provide something to suit all tastes. Of course, we hope our hints, tips and suggestions for alternatives will inspire you to adapt your own recipes and help you to expand your repertoire of brain-healthy meals.

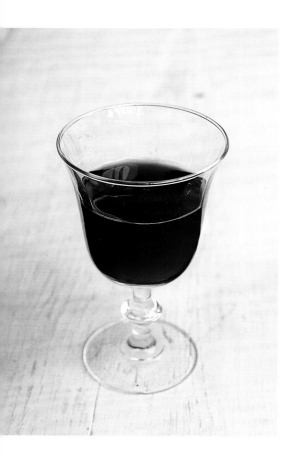

Alcohol in the brain-protective diet

Moderate alcohol intake may reduce the risk factors that lead to heart disease and stroke by increasing "good" HDL cholesterol and reducing the risk of blood clots forming. Alcohol may also contain neuroprotective nutrients, such as resveratrol in red wine (see page 20). A review of 33 key studies of the risks and/or benefits of alcohol consumption on MCI and dementia suggested that moderate alcohol intake might decrease the risk of heart disease and stroke and protect against cognitive decline and dementia, particularly in those who do not carry the ApoE ε4 gene. However, the authors were unable to reach a firm conclusion.

BE ALCOHOL AWARE

- Avoid frequent heavy or binge-drinking, which can harm health.
- Take a lead from the Mediterranean diet and consume alcohol mainly at mealtimes.
- If you don't drink alcohol there is no need to start for health reasons—the evidence for its benefits is not strong enough.

ALCOHOL GUIDELINES

Government guidelines

Government recommendations on safe drinking limits should be followed. Guidelines vary in each country but in the US, a standard drink is equal to 14 grams (0.6oz) of pure alcohol.

Alcohol limits: beer

This amount of pure alcohol is generally found in:
- 12 fl oz of regular beer (5% alcohol content)
- 8fl oz of malt liquor (7% alcohol content)

Alcohol limits: wine and spirits

It can also be found in:
- 5fl oz of wine (12% alcohol content)
- 1.5fl oz or a "shot" of 80-proof (40% alcohol content) distilled spirits or liquor (for example, gin, rum, tequila, vodka, whiskey).

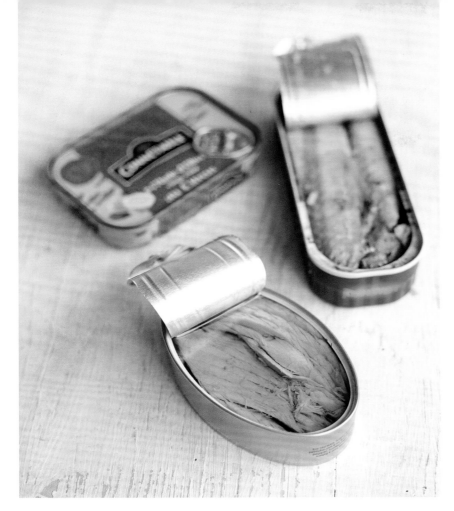

Nutrient analysis using food composition tables has limitations due to the natural variation in the nutrient composition of the foods themselves and as a result of variations in soil, agricultural methods, climate, transport, storage, and so on.

Due to the limited listing of foods in an appropriately cooked format on the databases, analysis was performed on raw ingredients to ensure consistency across all the recipes. Cooking methods and times may affect the retention value of some nutrients. Therefore nutrient values listed should be regarded as estimates only.

The number of fruit and vegetable portions is based on 80 grams (3 ounces) of raw fruit or vegetable (or 30 grams/ 1 ounce dried) and rounded to the nearest decimal. A recipe is defined as a "Source of" where the nutrient value for one portion is equal to or greater than 15 micrograms for selenium, 1.5 micrograms for vitamin D, 2 milligrams for vitamin E, 0.3 milligrams for B6, 33 micrograms for folate, 0.6 micrograms for B12 and 10 milligrams for vitamin C.

Notes on the nutritional analysis of recipes

Recipe analysis was completed in April 2014 using the Nutritics Professional Diet Analysis software. This uses the UK Composition of Foods Integrated Dataset (COFIDS) (including McCance and Widdowson 6th edition, and all its supplements), the Irish Foods Composition Database and a number of foods sourced by Nutritics based on user requests.

Weights of ingredients were based on those suggested by Nutritics (where available), sourced from textbooks and food surveys such as the National Diet and Nutrition Survey and the work of Wrieden and Barton (2005), or were estimated. Where more than one serving size was suggested, analysis was performed on the larger serving size.

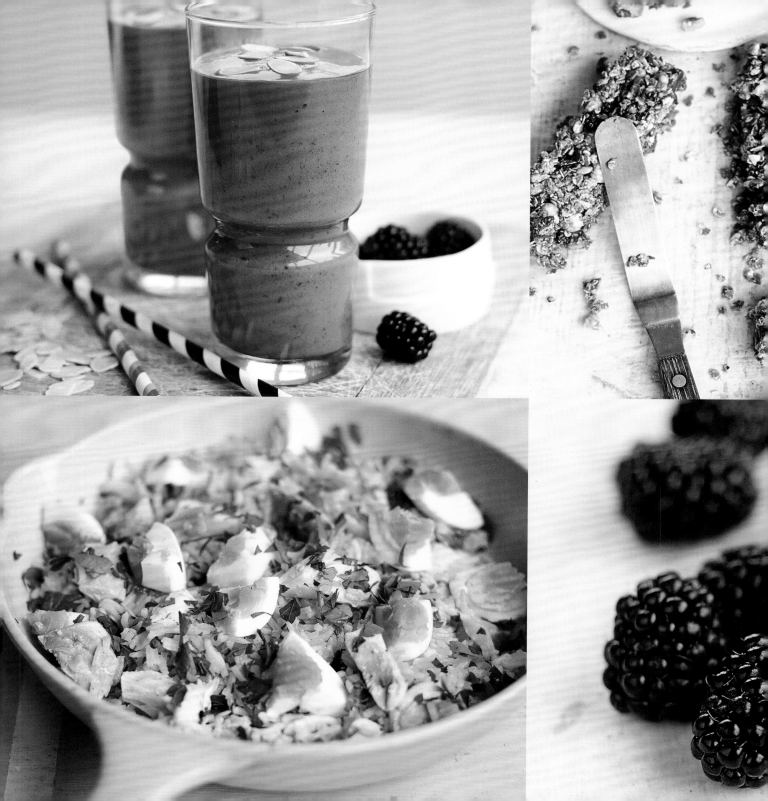

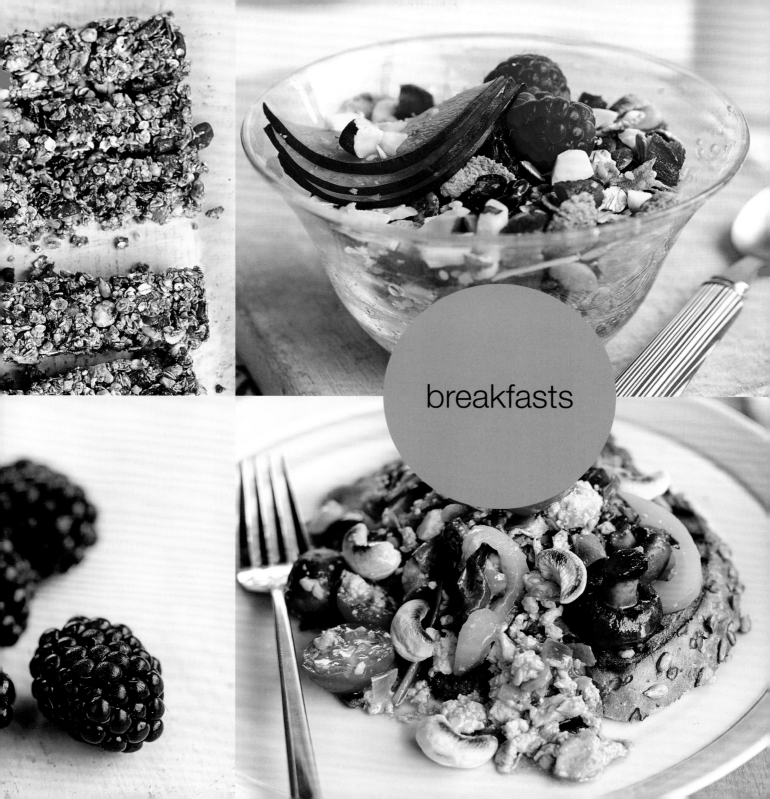

breakfasts

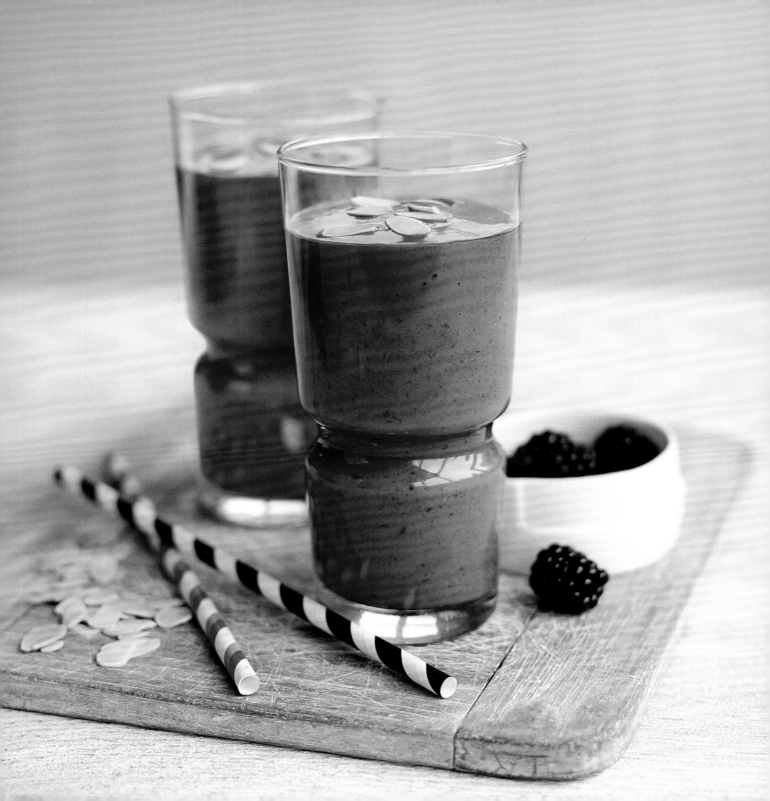

blackberry and almond smoothie

Quick and easy to make, this smoothie will give you a real nutrient boost to start your day.

SERVES 1

¾ cup blackberries
½ banana
½ cup soy yogurt or low-fat plain yogurt

2 teaspoons (about ¼ ounce) ground almonds
2 tablespoons skim or soy milk
Sliced almonds, to finish

Put the berries, banana, yogurt, ground almonds and a little of the milk in a tall jug and blend with a handheld blender until smooth.

Add more milk until the desired consistency is reached. Serve in a tall glass topped with a few sliced almonds.

Adding a tablespoon of rolled oats before blending will give a more textured smoothie. Other soft fruit or berries could be used instead of the blackberries.

Chosen as a source of: vitamins C, E, folate, soy, polyphenols / Per serving: 266 kcal; 11.2g fat; 1.2g saturated fat / 2 portions of fruit/vegetables

apple and spice oatmeal

This is a warming and easy-to-prepare breakfast and a great way to include fruit in the start to your day—or at any time.

SERVES 1

½ cup rolled oats
Scant ⅔ cup water
½ dessert apple, cored and cut into small bite-size pieces
Scant ½ cup soy milk

½ teaspoon ground cinnamon
Small pinch of salt
1 teaspoon sugar or honey (optional)
1 tablespoon sliced almonds

To prepare in the microwave:
Place all the ingredients except the almonds into a large heatproof bowl and microwave for approximately 3 minutes on high, stirring halfway through. Keep an eye on the oatmeal to ensure the mixture doesn't boil over.

To prepare on the stovetop:
Place all the ingredients except the almonds into a pan. Bring to a boil and simmer for 3–4 minutes, stirring continuously.

Remove from the heat and serve with the almonds sprinkled on the top.

Skim or low-fat milk could be used in place of the soy if preferred. You could also experiment with other fruit and nut/seed combinations, such as chopped dates or raisins and walnuts.

Chosen as a source of: vitamin E, folate, soy, polyphenols / Per serving: 304 kcal; 11.4g fat; 1.5g saturated fat / 0.5 portions of fruit/vegetables

granola breakfast pot

This delicious, nutritious breakfast combo has a good mix of flavors and textures and makes a great family breakfast as it can be adapted to taste. The granola on its own makes a great snack alternative to candy or chocolate bars.

MAKES ABOUT 6 SERVINGS

1 ounce Brazil nuts
1 ounce unsalted pistachios, shelled
1 tablespoon canola oil
3½ tablespoons honey
3 tablespoons water
½ ounce pumpkin seeds
½ ounce sunflower seeds

½ tablespoon sesame seeds
Generous ¾ cup jumbo oats

To serve (per person)
½ cup fat-free plain yogurt
1 portion (3 ounces) fresh or drained canned fruit such as banana, berries, apple, prunes

Preheat the oven to 300°F and line a large baking sheet with parchment paper. Chop the Brazil nuts and pistachios or blend briefly in a food-processor.

Put the canola oil, honey and water in a pan and heat gently until melted and well mixed.

Mix all the seeds and the oats in a large bowl, add the warmed liquid ingredients and stir together well. Spread the mixture across the baking sheet and bake in the oven until darkly golden—about 15–20 minutes. Keep an eye on the granola and check the oven regularly to avoid burning.

When ready, remove from the oven and allow to cool completely before storing in an airtight container. The granola will stay fresh for a couple of weeks.

To serve, place a portion of berries or chopped fruit in the base of a sundae dish, pour the yogurt on top and then sprinkle with a couple of handfuls of granola (about 1½ ounces).

Almonds work well in place of the Brazils or pistachios and will provide an extra boost of vitamin E.

Chosen as a source of: vitamins C, E, polyphenols / Per serving: 283 kcal; 11.6g fat; 1.9g saturated fat / 1 portion of fruit/vegetables

breakfast energy bars

The recipe for these bars was kindly provided by David Hill, Head Pastry Chef at the University of Surrey's Lakeside Restaurant. They are great for an energy-filled breakfast on the go and, as they contain no added fat, are much healthier than many store-bought bars.

MAKES 16 BARS

1¾ ounces whole hazelnuts, skin off
1¾ ounces whole almonds, skin off
1¾ ounces Brazil nuts
1¾ ounces unsalted pistachios, shelled
1¾ ounces dried figs, chopped
1¾ ounces currants
1¾ ounces dried cranberries

1¾ ounces dried apricots, chopped
1¾ ounces cocoa nibs or bittersweet chocolate chips
1 ounce pumpkin seeds
1 ounce sunflower seeds
1 cup rolled oats
1¼ cups rye flakes
1 tablespoon dark molasses
Scant 1 cup (7 ounces) honey

Preheat the oven to 325°F. Grease a 10½-inch square baking sheet and line with parchment paper. Roughly chop the nuts or blend very briefly in a food-processor.

Mix the chopped nuts with the rest of the dry ingredients in a large mixing bowl, then stir in the molasses and honey and mix until well combined.

Tip the sticky mixture onto the lined baking sheet and press down hard. This is easier if you lay a sheet of wax paper on top of the mix and press down with your hands before removing the paper.

Bake in the oven for 20–30 minutes until golden brown on top. Allow to cool on the baking sheet and when almost cold, cut into 16 portions. Store in an airtight container until required. The bars will keep well for several days.

These bars are high in calories so if you are watching your weight or prefer something a little less sweet, try using ¾ cup unsweetened apple juice and 2 tablespoons of honey instead of the cup of clear honey.

Chosen as a source of: vitamin E, polyphenols / Per bar: 228 kcal; 11.2g fat; 2.2g saturated fat / 0.5 portions of fruit/vegetables

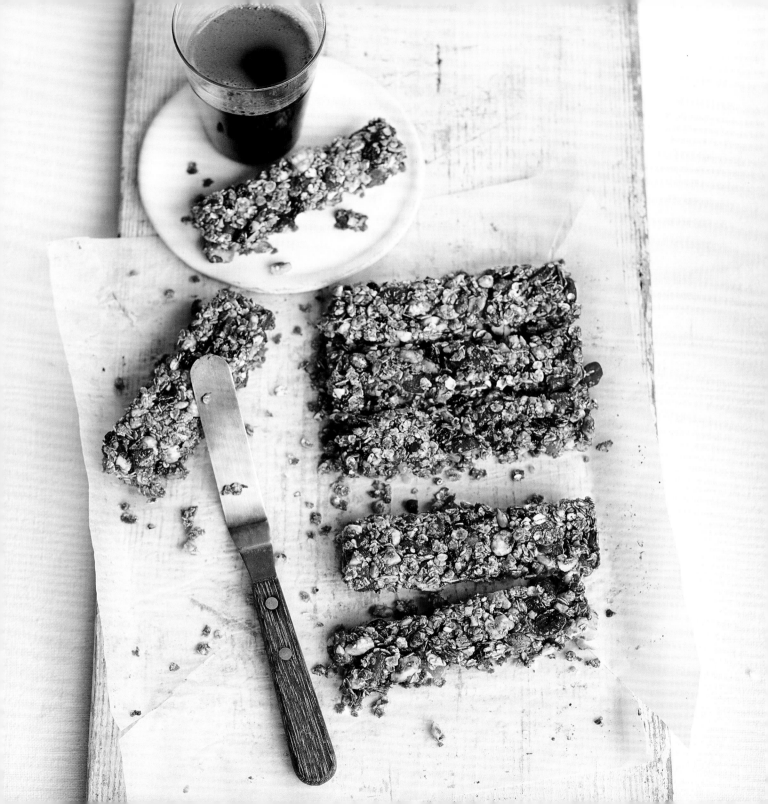

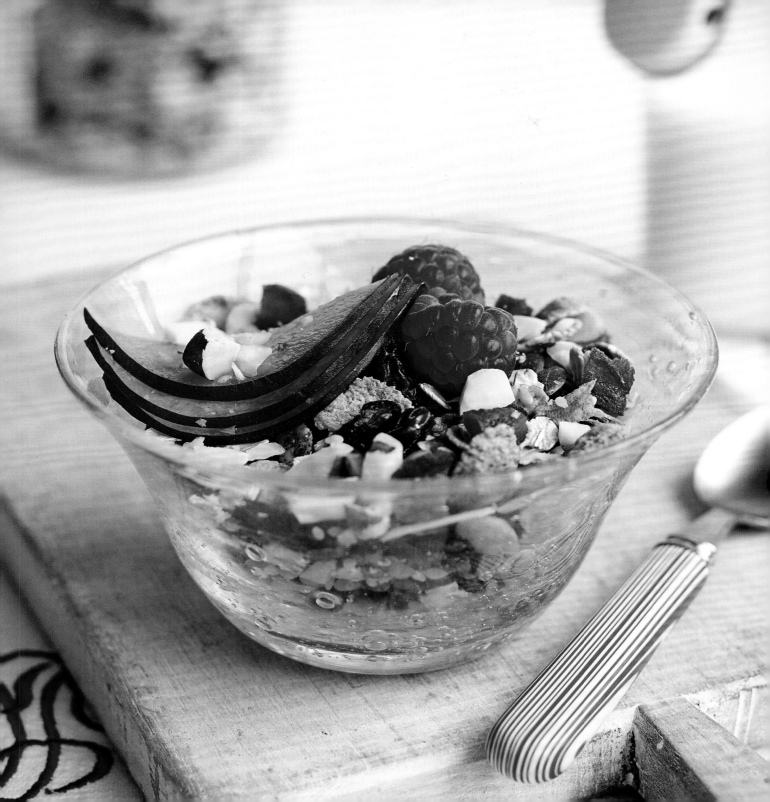

super muesli

Making your own muesli is easy and, while the ingredients in this recipe have been chosen to maximize beneficial nutrients, it's fine to adapt it to suit your own taste.

MAKES ABOUT 8 SERVINGS

2 heaped tablespoons each of:
Jumbo oats
Rye flakes (available from health stores)
Barley flakes (available from health stores)
Sliced almonds
Sunflower seeds
Pumpkin seeds
Golden flaxseeds
Sesame seeds
Raisins
Dried cranberries

To serve (per person)
2 Brazil nuts, chopped
2 ready-to-eat dried apricots, chopped
3 ounces berries (fresh or frozen), chopped apple or nectarine
Scant $2/3$ cup skim, rice or soy milk

Mix all the muesli ingredients together. Store in an airtight container away from direct sunlight until required.

One serving is about 1¾ ounces or 2 heaped tablespoons. Top with chopped Brazil nuts and apricots and fruit of your choice. Add milk and enjoy.

Choose fruit that is in season to maximize the flavor. Try serving with plain yogurt instead of milk.

Chosen as a source of: vitamins B6, B12, E, folate, selenium, soy, polyphenols / Per serving: 340 kcal; 16.2g fat; 3.1g saturated fat / 1.5 portions of fruit/vegetables

blueberry and wheatgerm pancakes

These light, fluffy pancakes are a great way to include fruit in your breakfast, and provide a boost of vitamin E from the wheatgerm.

SERVES 4

For the batter
2 free-range eggs
1 tablespoon canola oil
2 cups buttermilk
¾ cup wheatgerm
1½ cups all-purpose flour
1 tablespoon baking soda
Pinch of salt
1 cup fresh blueberries

For the sauce
1½ cups fresh blueberries
2 tablespoons water
2 teaspoons sugar

To make the batter, mix the eggs, oil and buttermilk in a medium bowl until well combined. Stir in the wheatgerm, flour, baking soda and salt and mix until blended. Fold in the cup of blueberries.

To make the sauce, place the 1½ cups of blueberries, water and sugar in a pan and simmer gently for 2–3 minutes, until the blueberries have broken down slightly and a sauce is formed. Set aside.

Place a large, nonstick frying pan over medium heat. Drop about 2 tablespoons of batter per pancake into the pan (depending on the size of your pan you may be able to cook 2 or more at once). When the top of the pancake starts to bubble, turn over and cook the other side. Repeat with the remaining batter. This recipe should make 10–12 pancakes—you can keep them warm in a low oven while cooking the others.

Serve immediately with the blueberry sauce.

Other soft fruits like strawberries or blackberries could also be used in place of the blueberries. If you can't get hold of buttermilk, low-fat plain yogurt diluted with a little water makes a good alternative.

Chosen as a source of: vitamins B6, B12, C, E, folate, polyphenols / Per serving: 299 kcal; 7.1g fat; 1.3g saturated fat / 1 portion of fruit/vegetables

scrambled eggs with smoked salmon

This is an easy way to include some fish in your diet. There is no need to add any salt as the smoked fish provides this.

SERVES 2

4 free-range eggs
3½ tablespoons skim milk
1 teaspoon olive oil or olive oil spread
2¼ ounces smoked salmon, torn
2 teaspoons fresh dill, roughly chopped
Freshly ground black pepper

Whisk together the eggs and milk and add pepper to taste.

Heat the olive oil in a nonstick pan over medium heat and pour in the egg mixture; leave to cook until the mixture appears slightly opaque.

Stir gently and repeat. While the egg mixture is still soft and runny, add the smoked salmon and dill and stir gently to incorporate. Continue to cook to your desired level of firmness and serve immediately.

Any type of smoked fish can be used and you can experiment with different herbs such as chives, fennel or parsley.

Chosen as a source of: vitamins B12, D, folate, selenium, MUFA, fish/seafood / Per serving: 217 kcal; 14.8g fat; 3.7g saturated fat

kedgeree

Kedgeree, an Indian-style breakfast, makes a wonderful brunch. This recipe uses salmon, but other fish like haddock would work just as well.

SERVES 4

14 ounces salmon fillets
1 tablespoon lemon juice
2 tablespoons and ½ teaspoon olive oil
3 free-range eggs
1½ cups basmati rice
½ red chili, chopped (or more to taste)
½ teaspoon turmeric
½ teaspoon garam masala
4 tablespoons freshly chopped flat-leaf parsley
Salt and freshly ground black pepper

Preheat the oven to 300°F.

Place the salmon fillets on a sheet of foil. Sprinkle with the lemon juice and ½ teaspoon olive oil and season with salt and pepper. Leave to rest for a few minutes then wrap the fish in the foil, place the package in a baking dish and cook for 15–20 minutes or until cooked through. Use a fork to break into large flakes.

Meanwhile, boil the eggs in water for 10 minutes until hard-boiled. Drain, peel and chop into ½–¾-inch pieces. Boil the rice for 10 minutes, or according to the package instructions. Drain and set aside.

Heat the 2 tablespoons olive oil in a pan and lightly stir-fry the chili for 30 seconds. Add the turmeric and stir for 1–2 minutes. Remove the pan from the heat, add the drained rice and stir through until the rice is a soft yellow color.

Gently fold in the flaked salmon, chopped egg, garam masala and most of the parsley. Scatter the remaining parsley over the top and serve.

You can cook the salmon the day before and keep in the refrigerator or even buy ready-poached salmon from the supermarket to reduce the preparation time.

Chosen as a source of: vitamins B6, B12, D, E, folate, selenium, MUFA, fish/seafood / Per serving: 547 kcal; 22g fat; 4g saturated fat

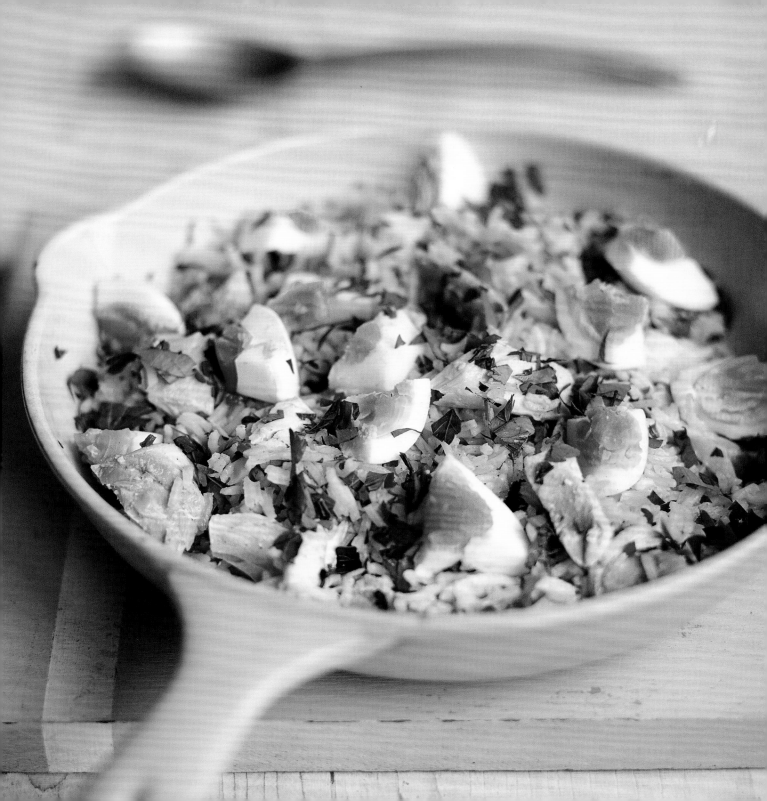

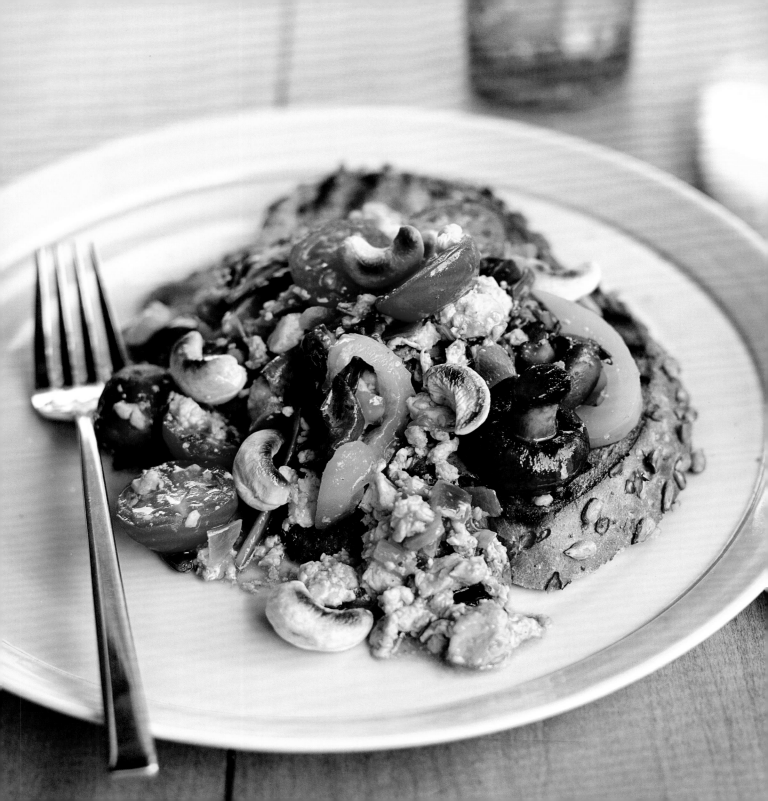

rainbow scrambled tofu

Thanks to Ilona and Adam Sharpe who developed this delicious breakfast/brunch dish as a vegan alternative to a full English breakfast. This brightly colored dish tastes as good as it looks!

SERVES 4 FOR BREAKFAST OR 2 FOR BRUNCH

½ cup unsalted cashews
1 tablespoon garlic-infused olive oil
1 red onion, finely chopped
10½ ounces silken tofu
1 teaspoon turmeric
1 tablespoon light soy sauce
1 tablespoon lemon juice
½ teaspoon dried mixed herbs
Pinch of chili flakes (or to taste)
3½ ounces baby button mushrooms
½ yellow pepper, sliced
3½ ounces cherry tomatoes, halved
2¾ ounces spinach leaves
Granary or wholegrain toast, to serve

Toast the cashews in a nonstick pan over medium heat until golden; put to one side.

Heat the garlic oil in a large, nonstick frying pan over medium heat. Add the chopped onion and cook gently until translucent, about 5 minutes. Add the tofu to the pan, breaking up gently with a spatula. Add the turmeric, soy sauce, lemon juice, dried herbs and chili flakes and stir gently. The tofu should now resemble scrambled egg.

Gently wash the mushrooms and add to the pan with the sliced pepper and cherry tomatoes. Cook gently until they are just tender, stirring occasionally. This will take about 5–10 minutes.

Tip the spinach into the pan, cover and leave for 2–3 minutes, after which time the leaves will have wilted and can easily be stirred into the tofu.

Serve on granary or wholegrain toast, topped with the toasted cashews.

If serving as a brunch, this also works well with vegetables such as broccoli, zucchini or even carrots, and with fresh bread instead of toast.

Source of legumes, soy and vitamin E / Per serving (based on 4 servings): 208 kcal; 14.6g fat; 2.5g saturated fat / 1.5 portions of fruit/vegetables

mushroom and tomato omelet

This omelet makes a warm and satisfying start to the day.

SERVES 1

½ tablespoon olive oil or olive oil spread
⅓ ounce chestnut mushrooms, washed and sliced
3 baby tomatoes, quartered
2 free-range eggs
1 tablespoon skim milk
Salt and freshly ground black pepper

Preheat the broiler to hot.

Heat the olive oil in a frying pan with a heatproof handle and sauté the mushrooms until golden brown. Add the tomatoes and sauté for a further 1–2 minutes.

Whisk the eggs with the milk and season with salt and pepper. Add the egg mixture to the mushrooms and tomatoes and stir gently.

Draw the set mixture from the sides of the frying pan into the middle and allow the liquid mixture to run to the sides. When the omelet has set, place the frying pan under the broiler to brown the top.

Chosen as a source of: vitamins B12, D, E, folate, MUFA, polyphenols / Per serving: 214 kcal; 17.4g fat; 3.9g saturated fat / 0.5 portions of fruit/vegetables

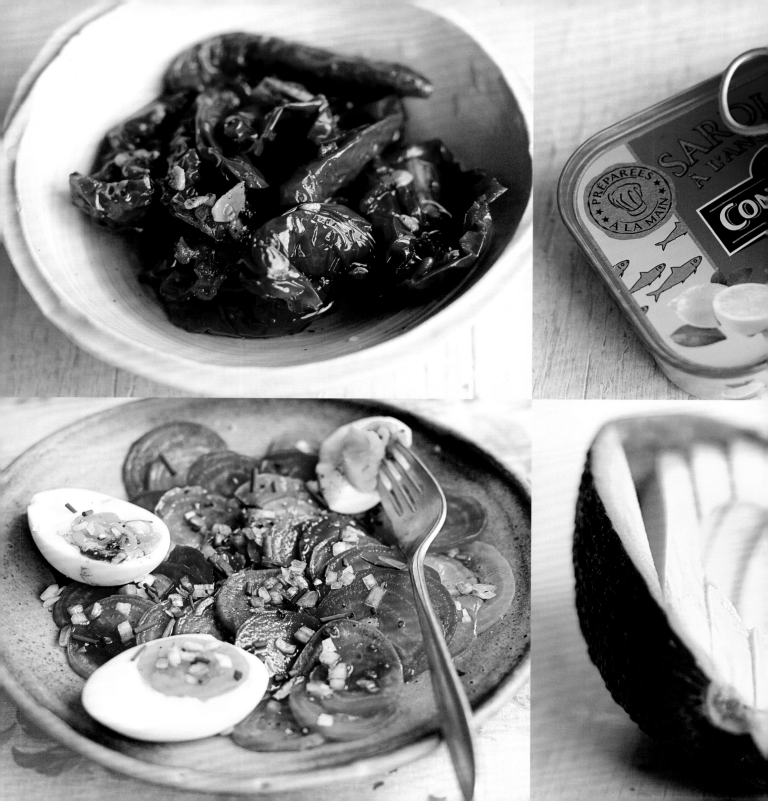

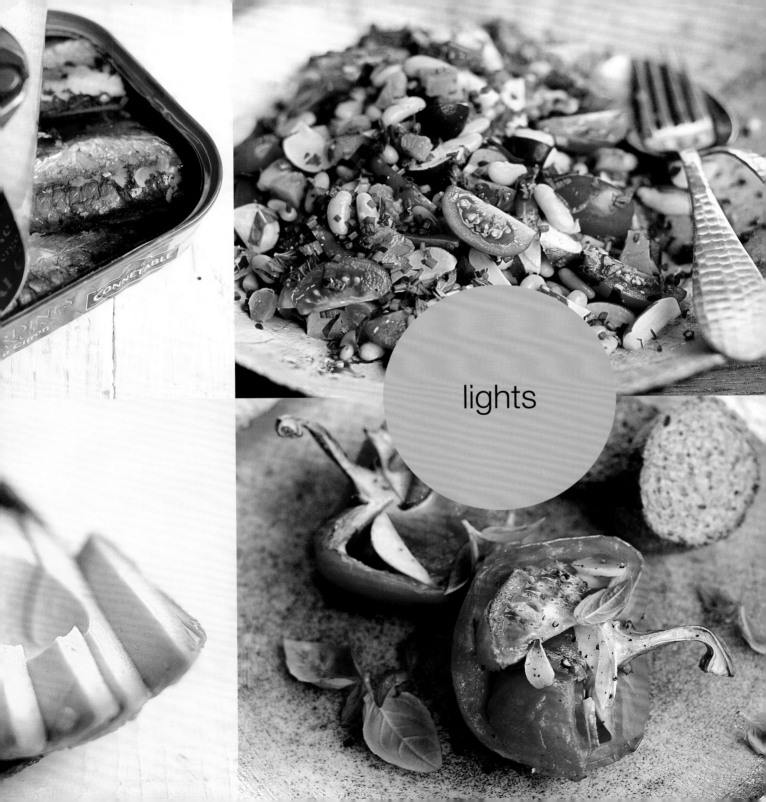

lights

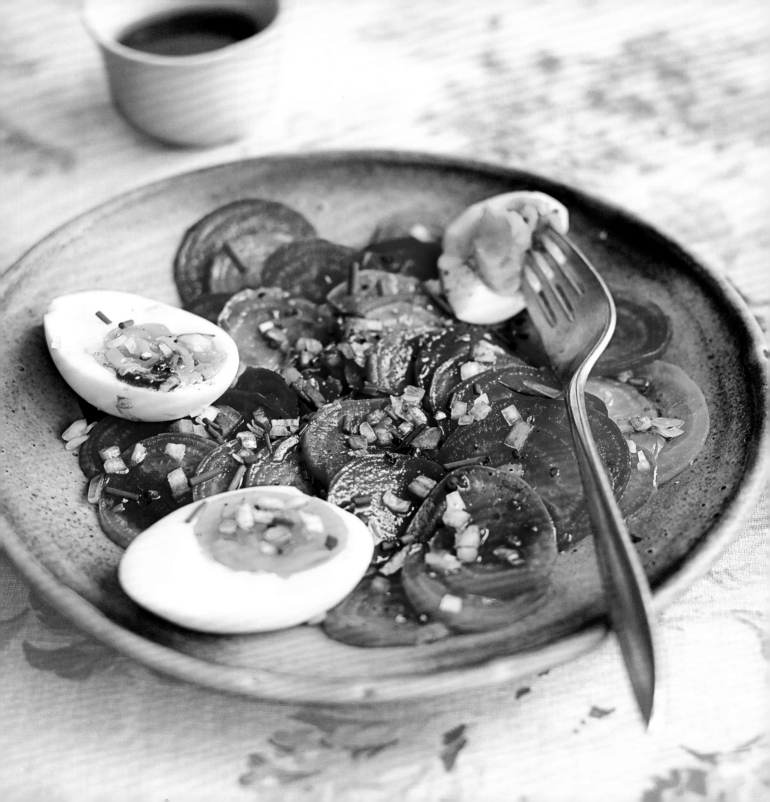

baby candy beet and soft-boiled egg salad

This recipe was kindly provided by John Walter, Head Chef and Restaurant Manager at the University of Surrey's Lakeside Restaurant. Here is what he had to say about it: "A favorite dish from my dear French mother-in-law's Brittany kitchen garden. A colorful, classic and delicious combination of earthy beets, shallots and eggs that is quick and easy to prepare."

SERVES 4

9-ounce selection of baby beets (try Chioggia, Golden and Cheltenham), washed
4 free-range eggs
1 large or 2 small shallots, finely chopped
A handful of freshly chopped flat-leaf parsley or chives

For the vinaigrette
1 small garlic clove, crushed
1 teaspoon smooth Dijon mustard
1 teaspoon honey
2 tablespoons balsamic or red wine vinegar
4 tablespoons walnut or canola oil
Salt and freshly ground black pepper

Bring a large pan of water to a boil and cook the beets for 40–50 minutes, depending on the size, or until they are soft. Alternatively, cook for 20 minutes in a pressure cooker. Allow to cool, then peel and dice or slice. Arrange in a serving dish.

Place the eggs in a pan of water and bring to a boil. Simmer for 5 minutes, then remove from the heat, run under cold water and peel. Carefully cut each egg in half and place around the cut beets. Scatter over the chopped shallot.

To make the vinaigrette, mix together the garlic, mustard, honey and vinegar in a small bowl. Whisk in the walnut or canola oil and season to taste.

Drizzle the vinaigrette over the salad, scatter over the parsley or chives and serve.

Chosen as a source of: vitamins B12, C, folate, polyphenols / Per serving: 225 kcal; 17.7g fat; 2.6g saturated fat / 1 portion of fruit/vegetables

hot beef and beet salad

A very quick and easy midweek supper. The combination of roasted beet, mustard dressing and peppery arugula gives it great depth of flavor.

SERVES 4

4–5 raw beets, peeled
2 red onions
1½ tablespoons olive oil
10½ ounces lean fillet or sirloin steak
3½ ounces arugula

For the dressing
3 tablespoons olive oil
1 tablespoon red wine vinegar
½ teaspoon wholegrain mustard

Preheat the oven to 350°F.

Combine all the dressing ingredients together and set aside.

Cut the beets into six wedges (or into quarters if they are small). Peel and cut the onions into six wedges, keeping the roots intact if possible, so that the wedges stay together. Place the beets and onions on a baking sheet and drizzle with 1 tablespoon of the olive oil. Bake for 25–30 minutes until crispy.

Place a griddle pan or frying pan over medium-high heat. Brush the steaks with the remaining ½ tablespoon of olive oil and fry for 3–4 minutes each side for a medium-rare steak (or until cooked to your preference). Remove from the heat and allow to rest for a minute.

Arrange the arugula leaves on a serving dish with the roasted beets and onions and drizzle with the dressing.

Cut the steak into thin slices and arrange on top of the salad. Serve immediately.

Chosen as a source of: vitamins B6, B12, folate, MUFA, polyphenols / Per serving: 277 kcal; 17.9g fat; 3.5g saturated fat / 1.5 portions of fruit/vegetables

eggplant and tomato gratin

The eggplant in this dish literally melts in your mouth and although the gratin tastes rich and indulgent it is actually extremely healthy. It keeps well in the refrigerator for several days and can be frozen and reheated successfully.

SERVES 4

2 medium eggplants, trimmed and cut into ½-inch slices
2 tablespoons olive oil
1 tablespoon freshly chopped thyme or oregano, or 1 teaspoon dried
1 quantity of Tasty Tomato Sauce (page 145)
1 ounce Parmesan cheese, coarsely grated
Freshly ground black pepper

Preheat the oven to 350°F.

Oil a baking sheet or line one with parchment paper. Arrange the eggplant slices in a single layer on the prepared sheet. Brush the top of the slices with the olive oil, saving enough to grease a shallow baking dish.

Bake the eggplant for about 10–15 minutes until slightly softened and just turning golden.

Arrange the baked eggplant in the base of the greased baking dish. Mix the thyme or oregano into the tomato sauce, season with black pepper and spread evenly over the eggplant. Sprinkle over the grated Parmesan and return to the oven for about 15–20 minutes until the top looks golden and crispy.

Serve with crusty bread and a green salad or with the Celery, Apple and Peanut Salad (page 138).

If you omit the Parmesan, this makes a delicious vegetable side dish. Vegetarians should use a vegetarian version of Parmesan and omit the anchovies from the tomato sauce.

Chosen as a source of: vitamin C, folate, polyphenols / Per serving: 135 kcal; 10.1g fat; 2.6g saturated fat / 2.5 portions of fruit/vegetables

lebanese salad

A lively, colorful and aromatic salad that makes a good side dish if you are having a barbecue.

SERVES 4

14-ounce can flageolet beans, drained
4¼ ounces radishes, quartered
2¾ ounces dried ready-to-eat apricots, roughly chopped
4¼ ounces baby plum tomatoes, quartered
½ red onion, finely chopped or 1½ ounces marinated red onion (see Warm Chicken and Pink Grapefruit Salad, page 74)
¾ ounce fresh mint, finely chopped
¾ ounce fresh flat-leaf parsley, finely chopped
¾ ounce fresh chives, snipped into short lengths
Zest and juice of 1 lemon
2 tablespoons basil-flavored olive oil
Salt and freshly ground black pepper

Combine all the ingredients in a large bowl and mix gently until well combined.

Taste and adjust the seasoning and then transfer the salad to a serving dish.

Adding some toasted cashews or almonds to the salad would make it a more substantial lunch or supper.

Chosen as a source of: vitamin C, folate, pulses, polyphenols / Per serving: 176 kcal; 7.4g fat; 1.1g saturated fat / 2.5 portions of fruit/vegetables

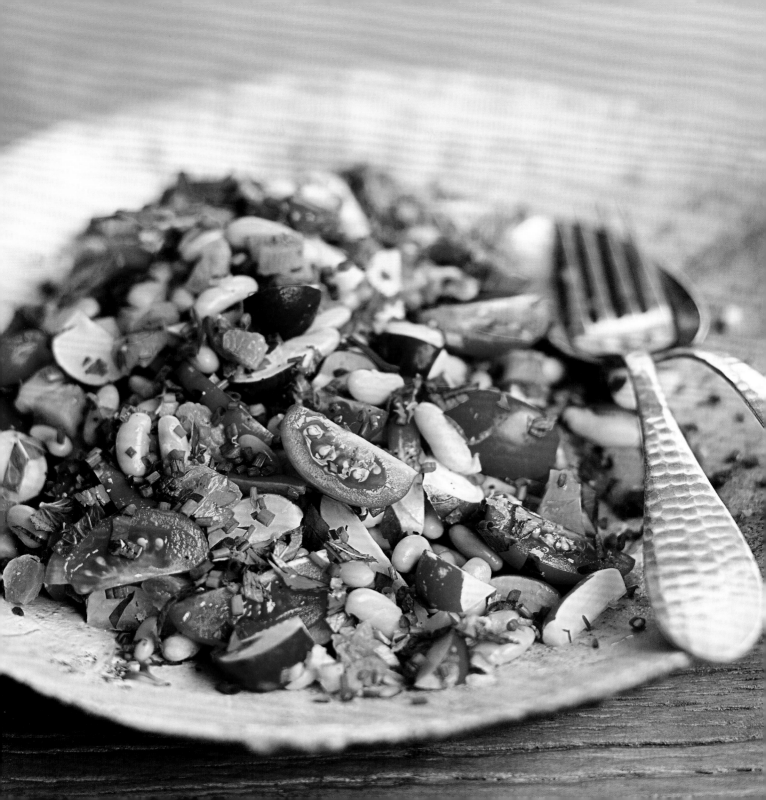

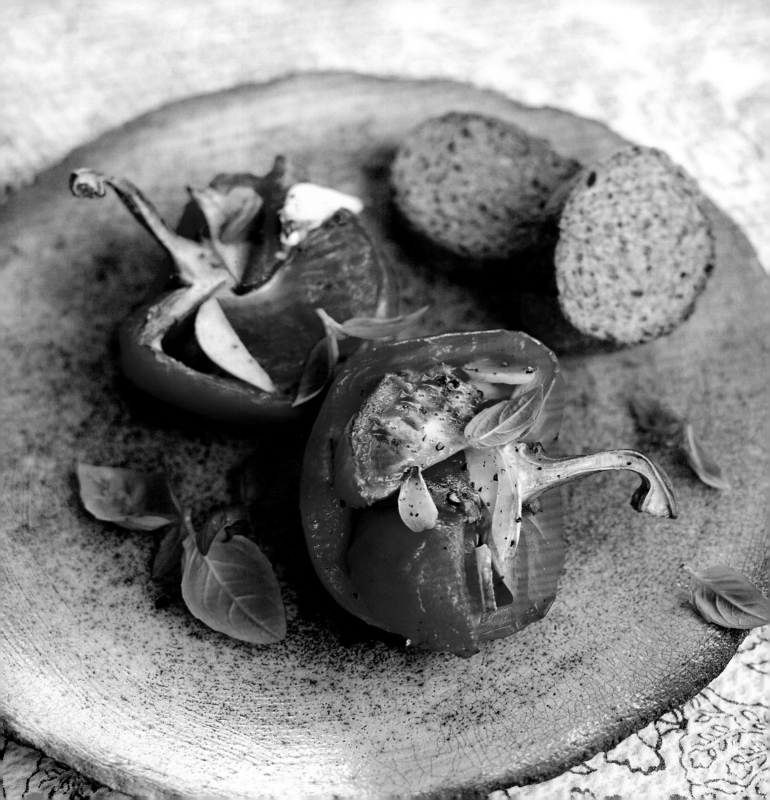

piedmont red peppers

This traditional Italian dish looks beautiful on the plate and makes a lovely appetizer or light lunch. The anchovies add depth and a good savory hit without imparting a fishy flavor.

SERVES 1

1 red pepper
1 tomato
2 canned anchovy fillets, drained and finely chopped
1 garlic clove, thinly sliced
1 teaspoon olive oil
A few basil leaves, roughly torn
Freshly ground black pepper

Preheat the oven to 350°F.

Cut the pepper in half, through the stalk if you can. Remove the seeds and pith but leave the stalks on. Arrange the pepper halves, cut side upward, in a lightly oiled, shallow baking dish.

Put the tomato in a heatproof bowl, cover with boiling water and leave for 1–2 minutes. Drain and peel off the skin, which will have started to separate from the flesh. Cut the tomato into quarters and place two quarters into the body of each pepper half.

Distribute the chopped anchovy fillets and sliced garlic evenly over the tomatoes. Drizzle with the olive oil and season with pepper (there is no need to add salt as the anchovies are salty enough).

Bake, uncovered, for 30–40 minutes. The peppers are ready when they are tender and slightly charred at the edges. Scatter over a few torn basil leaves and serve with some fresh bread to soak up the juices.

For vegetarians, omit the anchovies but add a splash of good-quality balsamic vinegar. If you are preparing these for a dinner party and don't know if your guests like anchovies, leave them whole and drape over the top so that your guests can remove them if wished.

Chosen as a source of: vitamins B6, B12, C, E, folate, fish/seafood, polyphenols / Per serving: 120 kcal; 5.7g fat; 0.9g saturated fat / 2 portions of fruit/vegetables

tortilla pizza

Using a tortilla for the base creates a lighter and healthier version of traditional pizza and can be ready in minutes. You can vary the topping to use whatever you have in the refrigerator. Thank you to Abigail Sharpe for sharing this recipe with us.

SERVES 1

1 tablespoon canola oil
1 ounce red pepper, seeded and chopped
1 ounce red onion, diced
1 ounce mushrooms, washed and sliced
A handful of spinach leaves
1 x 10-inch tortilla wrap, preferably wholewheat or multigrain
3½ ounces Tasty Tomato Sauce (page 145)
1 ounce low-fat Cheddar, grated
Large pinch of dried oregano
A few basil leaves, roughly torn

Preheat the oven to 350°F and line a baking sheet with parchment paper.

Heat the canola oil in a small frying pan over medium heat. Add the pepper, onion and mushrooms and fry gently for about 5 minutes until softened. Stir the spinach into the pan for 30 seconds or so until the leaves have wilted.

Place the tortilla on the lined baking sheet, spread the tomato sauce on top and sprinkle with the cheese and dried oregano.

Arrange the softened vegetables on top and bake for about 10 minutes until the cheese is melted and golden.

Add some torn basil leaves at the table and serve with a green salad.

Substitute low-fat mozzarella or feta for the Cheddar if you prefer. Note that if you have made the Tasty Tomato Sauce with anchovies, it will not be suitable for vegetarians.

Chosen as a source of: vitamins B6, C, E, folate, MUFA, polyphenols / Per serving: 441 kcal; 24g fat; 5.1g saturated fat / 2.5 portions of fruit/vegetables

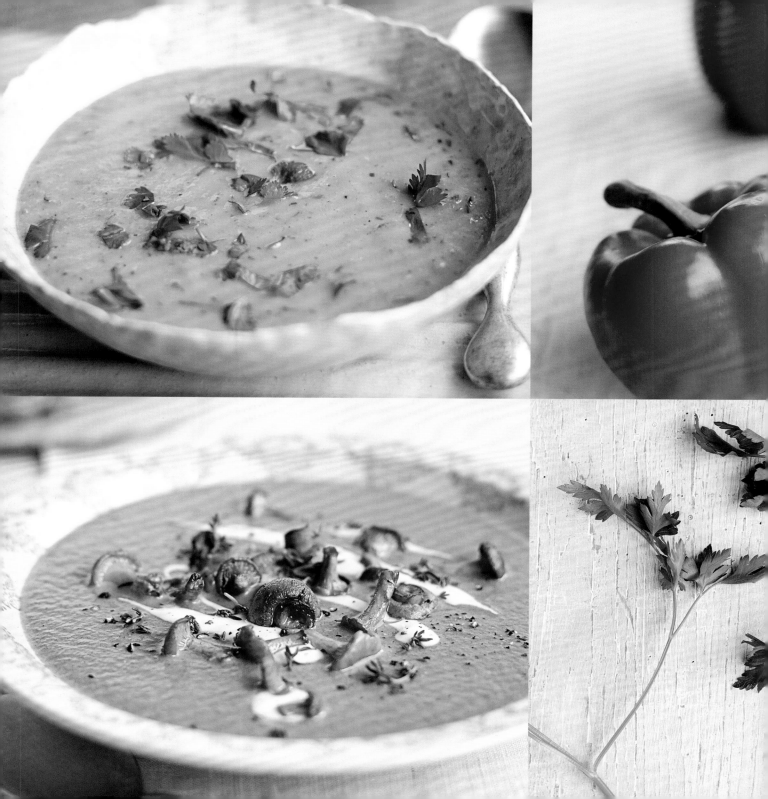

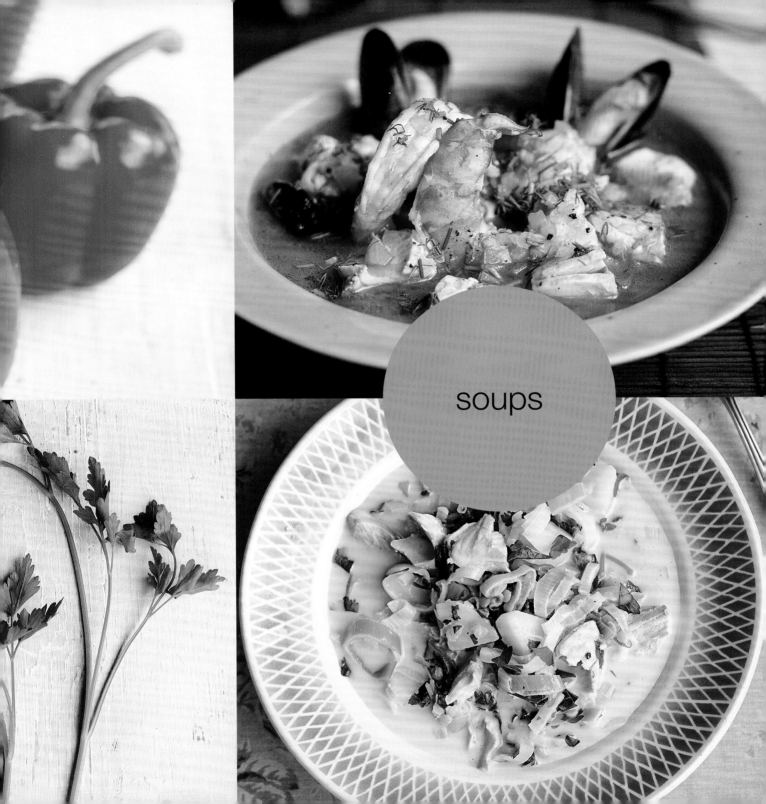

soups

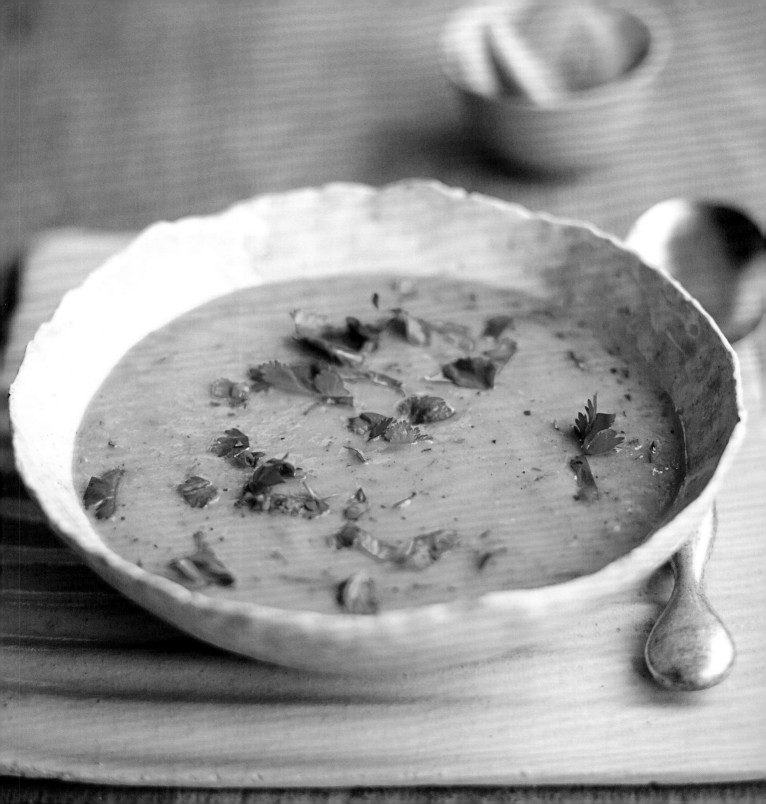

thai red lentil soup

Warming comfort food at its best. If you want to make the soup in advance it will keep in the refrigerator for several days and freezes well, but for the best flavor, add the lime zest and juice and the fresh herbs just before serving.

SERVES 6

1 tablespoon canola oil
1 large onion, chopped
2 sticks celery, chopped
2 carrots, diced
1 red chili, seeded and chopped (optional)
2 ounces (about ½ jar) red Thai curry paste
9 ounces (about 1½ cups) red lentils, rinsed and drained

2 zucchini (about 10½ ounces total), chopped
1¾ cups reduced-fat coconut milk
4¼ cups vegetable stock
Zest and juice of 1 lime
¾ ounce (about ¾ cup) freshly chopped flat-leaf parsley or cilantro
Salt and freshly ground black pepper

Heat the canola oil in a large pan over low-medium heat and add the onion, celery, carrots and chili, if using. Cook gently until softened, about 5–10 minutes. Add the red Thai curry paste and cook for about a minute, stirring occasionally.

Stir in the red lentils and then add the zucchini, coconut milk and stock. Bring to a boil then reduce the heat and simmer, covered, over low heat for about 30 minutes until the vegetables are tender and the lentils are very soft.

Allow to cool slightly, then blend until the consistency is to your liking. Stir in the lime zest and juice and the chopped herbs. Taste and adjust the seasoning and serve immediately.

Substitute other seasonal vegetables, such as green beans or broccoli, for the zucchini if you wish.

Chosen as a source of: vitamins B6, C, folate, pulses, polyphenols / Per serving: 256 kcal; 8g fat; 4.5g saturated fat / 2 portions of fruit/vegetables

cauliflower and cashew soup

This is a lovely "creamy" soup adapted from a recipe kindly provided by food blogger Monica Shaw of smarterfitter.com. Adding ground cashews to this soup helps to thicken it and imparts a lovely nutty flavor.

SERVES 4

2 tablespoons olive oil
1 onion, roughly chopped
2 garlic cloves
1 teaspoon cumin
1 cauliflower head (about 1¼ pounds), broken into florets
4¼ cups vegetable stock

A large handful of raw cashews, ground
Salt and freshly ground black pepper
A handful of toasted pumpkin seeds, to serve

Warm the olive oil in a heavy-based pan and cook the onion and garlic over medium heat until softened, about 5 minutes. Add the cumin and cook for a further minute.

Add the cauliflower and 3½ cups of the stock. Cover and simmer for 15–18 minutes until the cauliflower is tender.

Add the ground cashews and then, working in batches, puree the cooked cauliflower and cooking liquid using a handheld blender. Add the remaining stock, a little at a time, until the desired consistency is reached, then return to the pan and reheat gently.

Season with salt and pepper and serve garnished with the toasted pumpkin seeds.

Chosen as a source of: vitamins B6, C, folate, polyphenols / Per serving: 177 kcal; 10.7g fat; 1.8g saturated fat / 2.5 portions of fruit/vegetables

roasted butternut soup

This a very easy yet satisfying soup. Roasting the butternut enhances the flavors.

SERVES 4

1 medium butternut squash (about 1¾ pounds), peeled and seeded
1 onion, roughly chopped
2 garlic cloves, peeled
1½ tablespoons olive oil

4¼ cups hot vegetable stock
Salt and freshly ground black pepper
A handful of toasted pumpkin seeds, to serve

Preheat the oven to 350°F.

Cut the butternut squash into ¾–1¼-inch pieces and then tip onto a baking sheet with the onion and garlic cloves. Drizzle over the olive oil and toss to coat. Bake for 20–30 minutes until the butternut is soft.

Place the roasted vegetables into a food-processor or blender and add half the stock. Blend until smooth. Continue to add the remaining stock until the desired consistency is achieved.

Transfer to a pan to reheat gently, if necessary. Season with salt and pepper, sprinkle with some toasted pumpkin seeds and serve.

Replace the butternut squash with pumpkin or sweet potato, or a combination of both.

Chosen as a source of: vitamins B6, C, E, folate, polyphenols / Per serving: 151 kcal; 5.2g fat; 0.7g saturated fat / 3 portions of fruit/vegetables

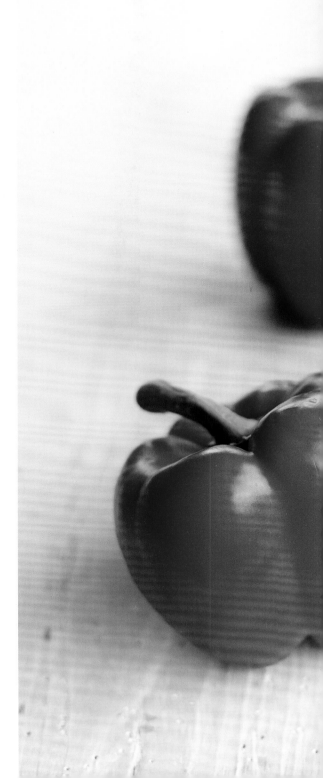

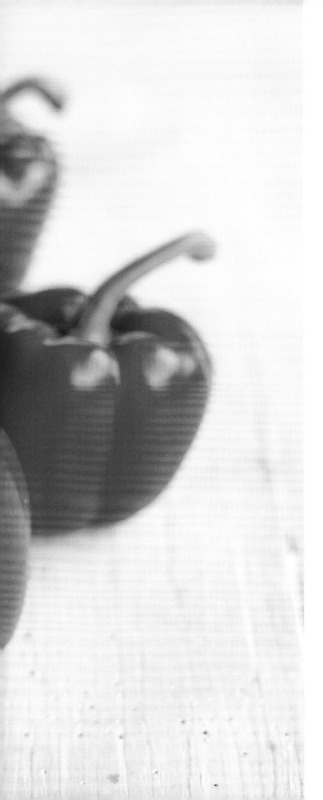

red vegetable soup

This vibrant soup is simple, quick to prepare, and very satisfying.

SERVES 4–6

1 tablespoon canola oil
1 large red pepper, seeded and roughly chopped
1 large red onion, roughly chopped
1–2 garlic cloves, crushed
14-ounce can chopped tomatoes
1 teaspoon dried oregano

½ x 14-ounce can red kidney beans, drained
4¼ cups vegetable stock
2 tablespoons Worcestershire sauce
1 ounce long-grain brown rice
¾ ounce fresh flat-leaf parsley, chopped

Heat the canola oil in a large pan over medium heat. Add the pepper, onion and garlic. Cover and cook gently for 5 minutes to soften.

Add the tomatoes, oregano, red kidney beans, stock, Worcestershire sauce and rice to the pan and stir. Bring to a boil then reduce the heat, cover, and simmer for about 20 minutes. Stir occasionally to prevent the rice from sticking. The soup is ready as soon as the rice is tender.

Stir through the chopped parsley. This soup is lovely served with crusty bread or garnished with toasted croutons.

Use mini wholegrain pasta shapes instead of rice if preferred.

Chosen as a source of: vitamins B6, C, E, folate, pulses, polyphenols / Per serving (based on 4 servings without bread or croutons): 198 kcal; 4.2g fat; 0.4g saturated fat / 3 portions of fruit/vegetables

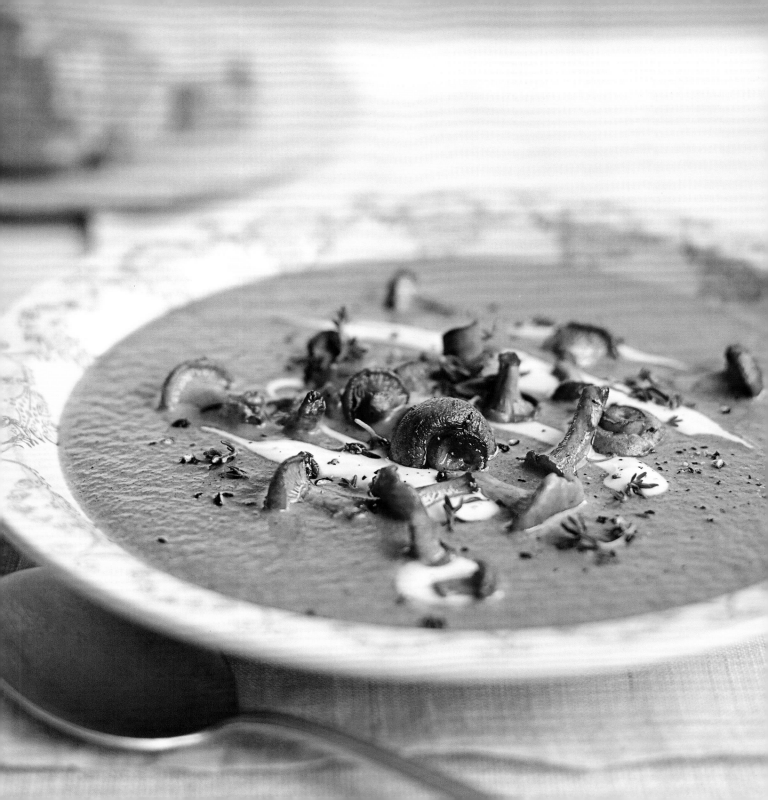

sun-dried mushroom soup

Sun-dried mushrooms provide an extra boost of vitamin D to this recipe. Topping the soup with whole roasted mushrooms adds texture and flavor.

SERVES 4

½ ounce dried wild mushrooms (preferably sun-dried)
1 tablespoon canola oil
2 sticks celery, chopped
1 large carrot, diced
1 leek, trimmed and thinly sliced
1½ ounces sun-dried tomatoes, finely chopped
1 teaspoon, plus a pinch of dried thyme
A few fresh thyme sprigs
Generous 2½ cups stock from a cube (vegetable, chicken or mushroom)

1¼ cups skim milk
12 ounces mixed fresh mushrooms, washed and chopped*
5½ ounces baby button mushrooms, washed*
1 tablespoon olive oil
Salt and freshly ground black pepper
Fresh thyme leaves and yogurt or cream, to garnish

see p.24 for how to increase the vitamin D content of mushrooms

Soak the dried mushrooms in ²/₃ cup of freshly boiled water for 15–20 minutes, then strain through a fine sieve, retaining the soaking liquid. Chop the mushrooms finely.

In a large pan, heat the canola oil over medium heat. Add the celery, carrot and leek and cook gently, covered, for 5–10 minutes or until beginning to soften. Add the chopped mixed fresh and wild mushrooms, sun-dried tomatoes, herbs, stock, milk and mushroom soaking liquid to the pan and bring to a boil. Simmer gently for 15 minutes.

Meanwhile, preheat the oven to 400ºF. Toss the baby mushrooms in the olive oil with a pinch of dried thyme and black pepper. Cook, on a baking sheet, for 15 minutes.

Alllow the soup to cool slightly before removing the thyme sprigs. Transfer to a food-processor or blender and blend until very smooth. Taste and adjust the seasoning. Top with the whole roasted baby mushrooms. Garnish with fresh thyme leaves and a drizzle of yogurt or cream.

Chosen as a source of: vitamins B6, B12, C, E, folate, selenium, polyphenols / Per serving: 171 kcal; 11.3g fat; 1.5g saturated fat / 3 portions of fruit/vegetables

creamy caraway and rosemary vegetable soup

The silken tofu in this aromatic soup gives it a smooth, creamy texture. The soup has a really luxurious feel, but isn't loaded with fat or calories. If you have broccoli stems left after making the Hearty Fish Pie (page 102), they can be used in this soup as they add loads of flavor.

SERVES 4–6

1 tablespoon canola oil
1 large onion, chopped
2 sticks celery, chopped
1 carrot, peeled and diced
1 garlic clove, crushed
1 tablespoon caraway seeds, bruised
1 tablespoon finely chopped rosemary
1 medium potato, peeled and diced

2–3 zucchini (about 14 ounces), trimmed and diced
7 ounces broccoli, stems and florets cut into small pieces
1 pound 5 ounces silken tofu
3½ cups vegetable stock
Salt and freshly ground black pepper

Heat the canola oil in a large pan over low heat. Add the onion, celery, carrot, garlic, caraway seeds and rosemary. Cook gently until the vegetables start to soften, about 10 minutes.

Stir in the potato, zucchini, broccoli and tofu, breaking up the tofu a little with a spatula. Add the stock and black pepper to taste. Bring to a boil, then reduce the heat and simmer for 15–20 minutes. At this point the tofu will give the soup a slightly curdled appearance but once it has been blended, this will turn to a luxurious creaminess.

Allow the soup to cool slightly then blend with a handheld blender until smooth and creamy. Taste and adjust the seasoning and serve.

Try making this soup with other vegetables that are in season. Silken tofu is a great alternative to cream—try it in other recipes.

Chosen as a source of vitamins B6, C, E, folate, selenium, soy, polyphenols / Per serving (based on 4 servings): 277 kcal; 12g fat; 1.5g saturated fat / 3.5 portions of fruit/vegetables

tuscan bean soup

There are numerous variations on this rustic Italian soup but this version is particularly flavorful and colorful—a real crowd pleaser.

SERVES 4–6

1 tablespoon canola oil
1 large leek, cleaned and thinly sliced
1 red onion, chopped
1 large orange pepper, seeded and sliced
7 ounces savoy cabbage, shredded
14-ounce can chopped tomatoes

14-ounce can mixed beans, drained
2 tablespoons tomato paste
1 tablespoon black olive pesto
1 lemon, cut into wedges
5 cups vegetable stock
2 teaspoons dried mixed herbs
3½ ounces chestnut mushrooms, washed and thickly sliced

Heat the canola oil in a large pan over medium heat. Add the leek and onion. Reduce the heat, cover and leave to soften for 5–10 minutes.

Add all the other ingredients except the mushrooms to the pan, bring to a boil and simmer, covered, for 15 minutes. Add the mushrooms and simmer for a further 10 minutes.

Remove the lemon wedges from the pan and serve the soup with chunks of crusty bread.

You can use any canned beans, such as cannellini, borlotti or lima beans for this soup.

Chosen as a source of: vitamins B6, C, E, folate, pulses, polyphenols / Per serving (based on 4 servings): 143 kcal; 1.7g fat; 0.3g saturated fat / 4.5 portions of fruit/vegetables

salmon and watercress chowder

This is a chunky main course soup perfect for a filling lunch.

SERVES 4

9 ounces salmon fillets
3 cups skim milk
2 thyme sprigs
3 cups vegetable stock
2 leeks, washed and thinly sliced
1 large potato, peeled and diced

2¾ ounces (about ½ cup) red lentils, rinsed and drained
2¾ ounces fresh flat-leaf parsley, chopped
2 ounces watercress, finely chopped
Salt and freshly ground black pepper

Place the salmon fillets in a frying pan with the milk and thyme sprigs. Gradually bring to a boil, then reduce the heat and poach the fish for 2–4 minutes. Remove the salmon with a slotted spoon and set aside.

Transfer the poaching liquid and herbs to a large pan and add the stock, leeks, potato and lentils. Bring to a boil then reduce the heat and simmer, covered, for about 30 minutes until the potato is cooked and the lentils are very soft.

Roughly flake the cooked salmon and stir into the chowder with the parsley and watercress. Season to taste with salt and pepper.

For a vegetarian version of the chowder, replace the poached salmon with a 14-ounce can of lima beans (drained).

Chosen as a source of: vitamins B6, B12, C, D, E, folate, selenium, fish/seafood, pulses, polyphenols / Per serving: 311 kcal; 8.8g fat; 1.6g saturated fat / 1.5 portions of fruit/vegetables

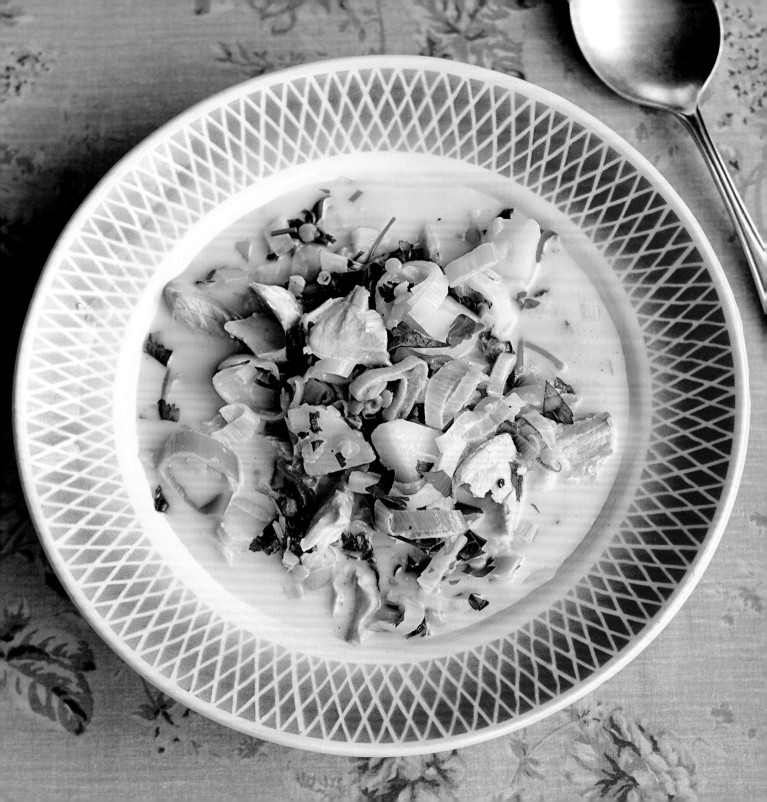

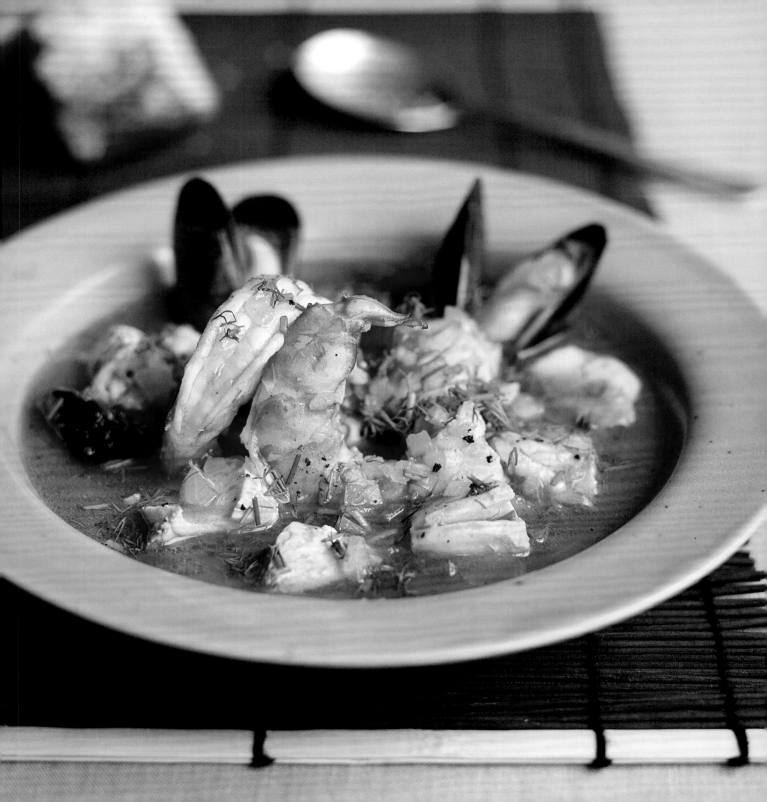

indonesian tofu and shrimp soup

This zingy, oriental soup is packed with bold, fresh flavors that complement one another beautifully.

SERVES 4–6

1 tablespoon canola oil
Zest and juice of 1 lime
1 red onion, chopped
1–2 garlic cloves, crushed
1 green chili, seeded and
   finely chopped
2-inch piece of fresh ginger,
   peeled and grated
1 teaspoon ground coriander
Scant 1 cup low-fat coconut
   milk
Scant 4 cups boiling water

1 tablespoon tahini
1 tablespoon peanut butter
Juice of 1 lemon
3½ ounces smoked tofu, cubed
3½ ounces frozen peas
7 ounces raw shrimp
2¾ ounces green tea noodles,
   broken into ¾-inch lengths
5½ ounces spinach
1/3 ounce chives, snipped
Salt and freshly ground black
   pepper

Heat the canola oil in a large pan over medium heat. Add the lime zest, onion, garlic, chili and ginger and cook gently until softened. Add the coriander and cook for 1–2 minutes, stirring frequently. If the mixture seems to be sticking to the pan, add a little water.

Add the coconut milk, boiling water, tahini, peanut butter and lemon juice to the pan. Bring to a boil, stirring well to dissolve the peanut butter and tahini, then reduce the heat and simmer for 5 minutes.

Add the tofu, peas, shrimp and noodles to the soup and simmer for 5 minutes until the noodles and shrimp are just cooked. Add the spinach to the pan, cover and leave for 2 minutes for the leaves to wilt, then stir through the soup.

Add a good grinding of black pepper and salt as required. Stir in the lime juice and serve garnished with chopped chives.

If using cooked shrimp, add them to the soup with the spinach for the last 2 minutes of cooking. Green tea noodles are available in oriental supermarkets but if you can't get hold of them, udon or rice noodles also work well.

Chosen as a source of: vitamins B12, C, E, folate, fish/seafood, soy, pulses, polyphenols / Per serving (based on 4 servings): 271 kcal; 13.5g fat; 4.5g saturated fat /1 portion of fruit/vegetables

spiced fish soup

You can adapt this spicy, flavorful soup to use any fairly firm fish. Ask your fishmonger what is best on the day—or you could use one of the fresh or frozen fish combination packs often sold in supermarkets.

SERVES 4

2 tablespoons olive oil
1 onion, finely chopped
2 garlic cloves, crushed or
   finely chopped
1 celery stick, finely chopped
1 carrot, finely chopped
1 teaspoon paprika
½ cup dry white wine
14-ounce can chopped
   tomatoes
4¼ cups good-quality fish stock
14 ounces mixed cod, salmon
   and haddock, skinned and
   cut into large cubes

12 mussels, washed and
   debearded (discard any open
   mussels that do not close
   when tapped sharply)
1 teaspoon dried dill or 1
   tablespoon fresh dill
12 shrimp, peeled and
   deveined
Salt and freshly ground black
   pepper

Heat the oil in a pan and cook the onion, garlic, celery and carrot over medium heat until just soft. Add the paprika and cook for a further minute.

Add the wine, bring to a boil and reduce for 1–2 minutes. Add the tomatoes and the stock, then return to a boil and simmer for 20 minutes.

Add the cubed fish, mussels and dill and simmer for 1 minute. Then add the shrimp and simmer for another 2 minutes until the mussels have opened. Discard any mussels that remain closed.

Season to taste with salt and pepper and serve with crusty wholewheat bread.

Chosen as a source of: vitamins B6, B12, C, D, E, folate, selenium, fish/seafood, polyphenols / Per serving: 306 kcal; 12.2g fat; 2g saturated fat / 2 portions of fruit/vegetables

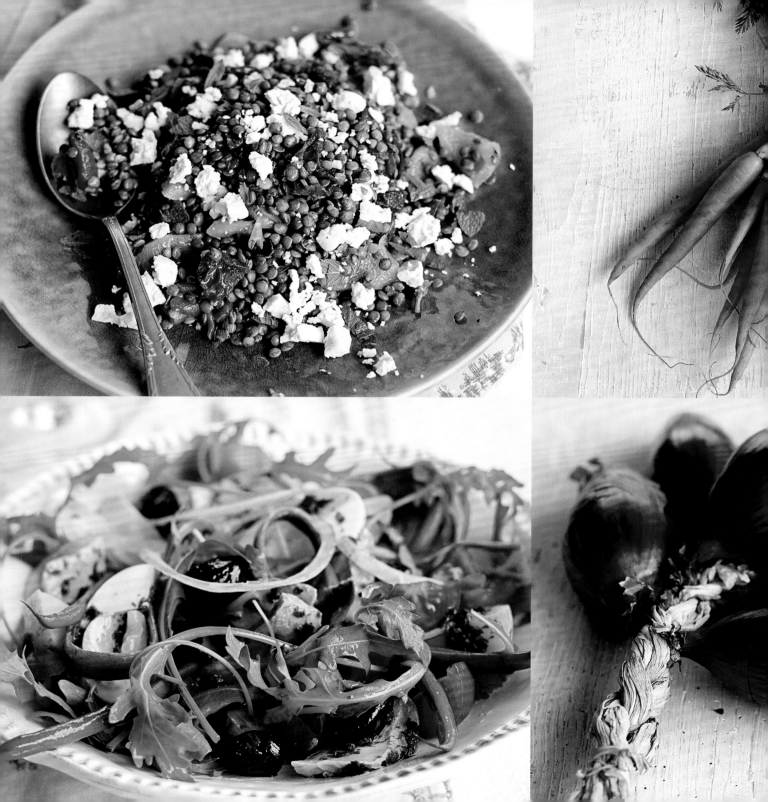

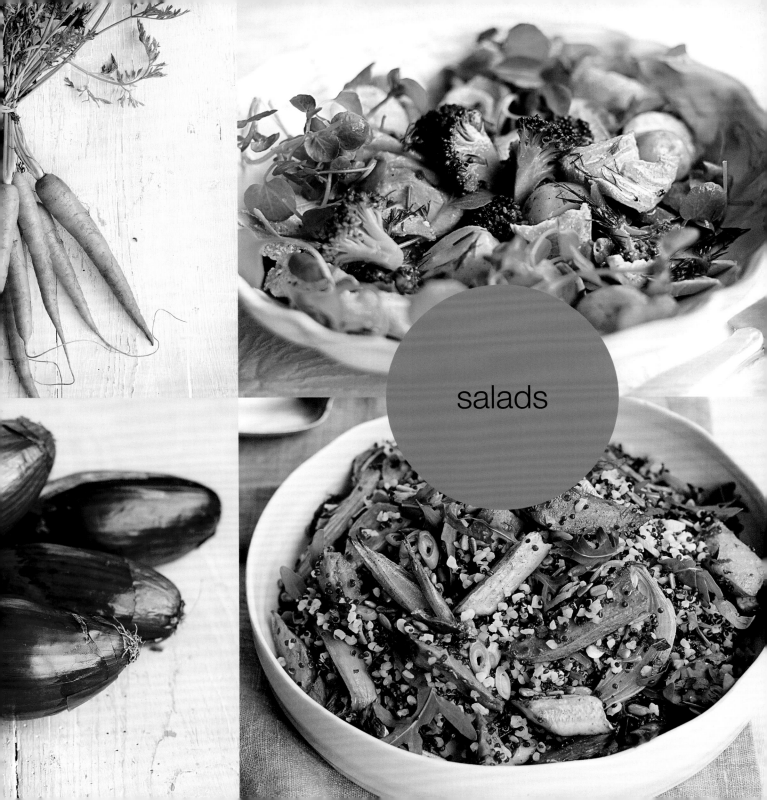

salads

asian peanut and pink grapefruit salad

This uses many of the same ingredients as the Warm Chicken and Pink Grapefruit Salad (opposite) but is suitable for vegetarians and provides a totally different taste thanks to the use of Asian flavors in the dressing.

SERVES 2 AS A MAIN COURSE OR 4 AS AN APPETIZER

1 large red onion, very thinly sliced
Scant $^2/_3$ cup white wine vinegar
3½ ounces sugar
2 little gem lettuces
2 ounces watercress
4-inch chunk of cucumber, thickly sliced
1 pink grapefruit, peel and pith removed, cut into segments
2¾ ounces dry-roasted peanuts

For the dressing
1 teaspoon palm sugar
1 teaspoon fish sauce
Juice and zest of ½ lime
2 teaspoons chopped fresh mint
½ red or green chili, seeded and finely chopped
2 teaspoons finely chopped shallot
2 teaspoons sesame oil

Place the sliced red onion in a small heatproof bowl. Put the white wine vinegar and sugar in a small pan and heat gently, stirring occasionally, until the sugar dissolves. Increase the heat and bring to a boil.

Pour the sweetened vinegar over the onions and leave to marinate for 10–60 minutes. Marinating the onions takes away their rawness, adds a subtle sweetness and turns them a pretty pink color. The longer you leave them, the more their flavor will change.

Separate the lettuce leaves and place in a large bowl with the watercress and cucumber. Combine the dressing ingredients in a screw-top jar, shake well, then pour over the cucumber and leaves and toss well to combine.

Arrange the dressed salad on a serving dish, arrange the grapefruit segments on top and scatter over the peanuts. Drain the marinated onion and arrange on top of the salad.

Chosen as a source of: vitamins B6, C, folate, MUFA, pulses, polyphenols / Per serving (based on serving 2): 376 kcal; 25g fat; 4.3g saturated fat / 4 portions of fruit/vegetables

warm chicken and pink grapefruit salad

Pink grapefruit is an underused ingredient but its interesting sweet/sour flavor works well with chicken. The marinated red onion is key and makes this a really memorable dish with great flavor and texture. Pictured right.

SERVES 2 AS A MAIN COURSE OR 4 AS AN APPETIZER

1 large red onion, very thinly sliced
Scant $^2/_3$ cup white wine vinegar
3½ ounces sugar
2 little gem lettuces
2 ounces watercress
1 tablespoon olive oil
7 ounces cooked chicken, roughly shredded

1 pink grapefruit, peel and pith removed, cut into segments

For the dressing
2 tablespoons extra virgin olive oil
2 teaspoons white wine vinegar
1 heaped teaspoon grain mustard
1 teaspoon honey

To make the marinated red onion, follow the first two steps of the recipe on the left for the Asian Peanut and Pink Grapefruit Salad.

Separate the lettuce leaves and place in a large bowl with the watercress. Combine the dressing ingredients in a screw-top jar, shake well then pour over the cucumber and leaves and toss well to combine.

Then, in a nonstick pan, heat a tablespoon of olive oil until very hot. Add the shredded chicken meat to the pan, leave for 2 minutes until starting to crisp up, then turn once or twice until it is golden and crispy.

On a serving dish, arrange the dressed leaves, grapefruit segments and crispy chicken and top with the drained marinated onions.

This salad would be a good way to use up leftover Thanksgiving turkey instead of chicken.

Chosen as a source of: vitamins B6, C, E, folate, selenium, MUFA, polyphenols / Per serving (based on serving 2): 406 kcal; 23g fat; 3.5g saturated fat / 3.5 portions of fruit/vegetables

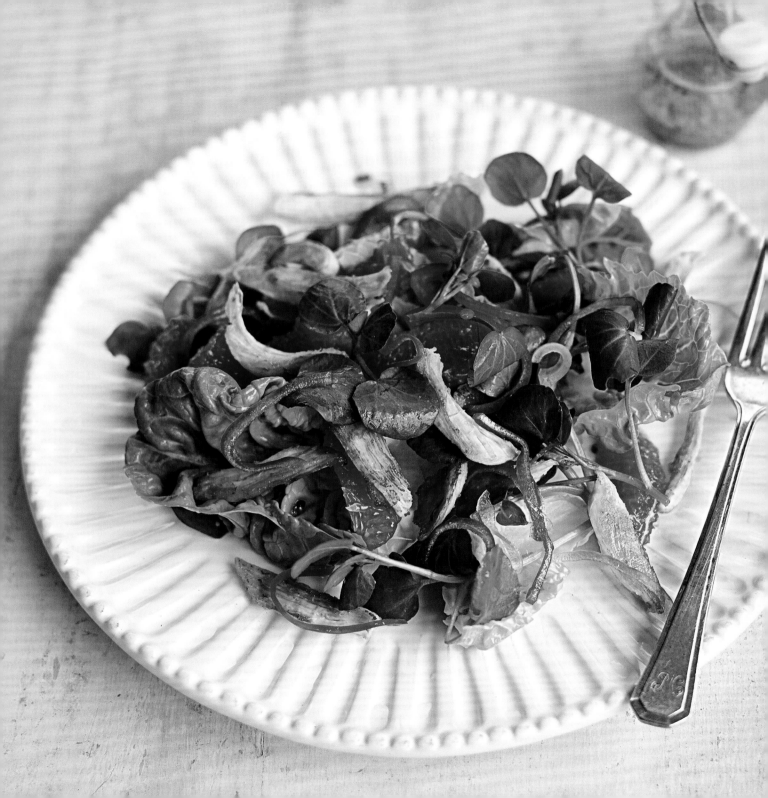

greek salad

This variation on a traditional recipe includes grapes, which make the salad lighter and more colorful. They also add an interesting flavor to complement the saltiness of the olives and feta.

SERVES 2–4

2 little gem lettuces or
  1 romaine lettuce
1¾ ounces arugula leaves
½ cucumber
7 ounces baby plum tomatoes,
  halved
5½ ounces red seedless
  grapes, halved
5½ ounces low-fat feta cheese

2¾ ounces (about ¾ cup) pitted
  black or Kalamata olives,
  halved
½ small red onion, finely
  chopped
¾ ounce fresh mint, chopped
1 tablespoon olive oil
Zest and juice of 1 lemon
Freshly ground black pepper

Break the lettuce into individual leaves and arrange on a serving dish. Scatter the arugula leaves on top.

Cut the cucumber in half lengthwise and then remove the seeds with a spoon. Cut each half lengthwise again and then cut into chunks. Place in a large bowl.

Add the remaining ingredients to the bowl and mix gently until well combined.

Pile the contents of the bowl on top of the lettuce and arugula and serve with crusty bread.

Try using a flavored olive oil such as basil or chili.

Chosen as a source of: vitamins, C, E, folate, MUFA, polyphenols / Per serving (based on serving 4) (not including bread): 199 kcal; 13.8g fat; 4g saturated fat / 2 portions of fruit/vegetables

french lentil salad with goat cheese

Make sure you use authentic French (Puy) lentils for this recipe. They have a distinctive peppery taste and a wonderful, dark, green-black color. The contrast of flavors and textures make this salad stand out. It can be served warm or cold.

SERVES 4

9 ounces (about 1½ cups)
  French lentils, washed and
  drained
Zest and juice of 1 lemon
1 tablespoon olive oil
1¾ ounces sun-dried tomatoes,
  drained and chopped

1¾ ounces chargrilled peppers
  in olive oil, drained and
  chopped
¾ ounce fresh mint, roughly
  chopped
1¾ ounces goat cheese,
  crumbled

Place the lentils in a medium pan with the lemon zest. Cover with about twice their volume of water and bring to a boil. Cover the pan, lower the heat and simmer for 15–18 minutes until *al dente*.

Drain the lentils, transfer to a serving dish and mix immediately with the lemon juice and olive oil. Stir through the tomatoes and peppers.

Allow the salad to cool a little before stirring in the chopped mint and topping with crumbled goat cheese. Don't add the mint too soon or the heat from the lentils will turn it black.

Serve warm or cold.

If you leave out the goat cheese, this salad would make a delicious accompaniment to most types of white or oily fish.

Chosen as a source of: vitamins B6, C, E, folate, selenium, pulses, polyphenols / Per serving: 314 kcal; 13.3g fat; 3.1g saturated fat / 1 portion of fruit/vegetables

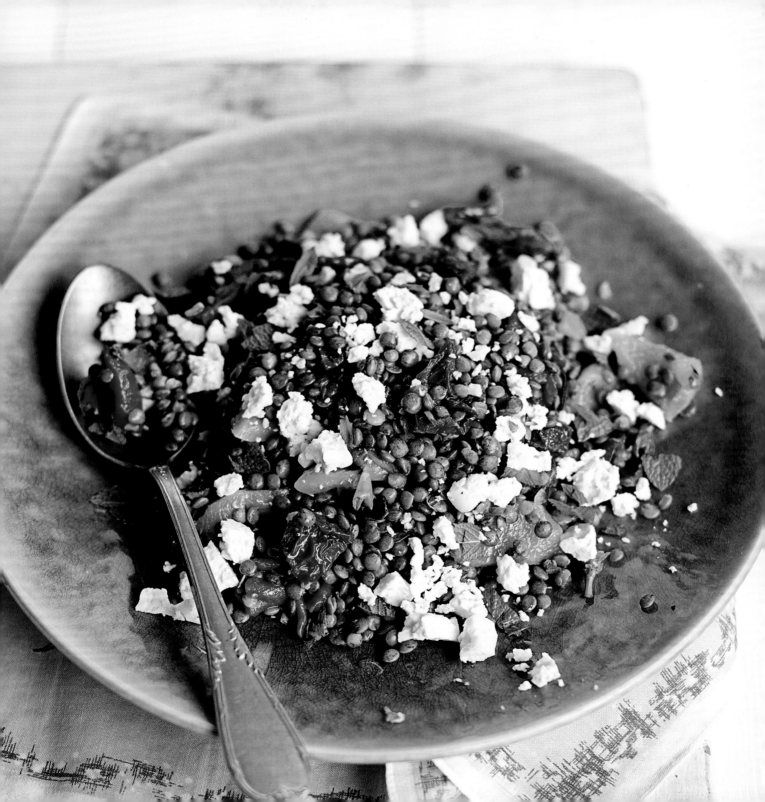

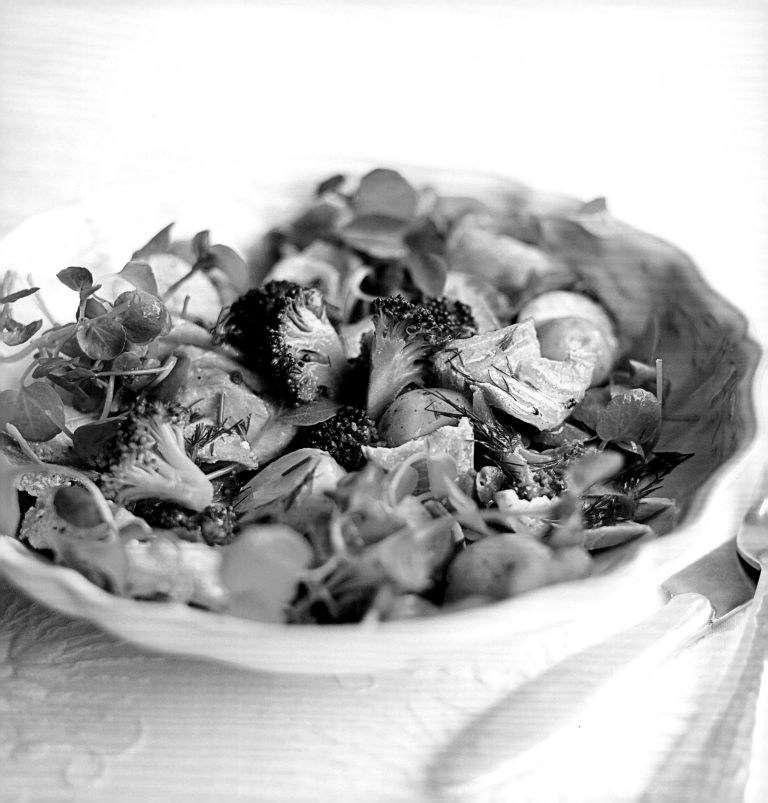

salmon and watercress salad

Combining salmon with the peppery taste of watercress makes a very tasty and satisfying meal. Fresh or canned salmon can be used as both are rich in long-chain omega-3 fats.

SERVES 2

5½ ounces baby new potatoes (2–3 per person)	**For the dressing**
2¾ ounces broccoli	3 tablespoons olive oil
2¾ ounces watercress, washed and dried	1 tablespoon lemon juice
	1 teaspoon mustard
2 cooked salmon fillets, flaked, or 7 ounces canned salmon	1 tablespoon chopped fresh dill
	1 teaspoon honey

Whisk together all the dressing ingredients until well combined and set aside.

Boil the baby potatoes for about 10 minutes or until just cooked, adding the broccoli for the last 1–2 minutes (you want it just tender, not overcooked). Drain and when cool enough to handle, slice the potatoes.

To assemble, place the watercress in a serving dish, add the salmon, potatoes and broccoli and drizzle with the dressing.

Use asparagus, when in season, to replace or complement the broccoli.

Chosen as a source of: vitamins B6, B12, C, D, E, folate, selenium, MUFA, fish/seafood, polyphenols / Per serving: 442 kcal; 31g fat; 4.9g saturated fat / 1 portion of fruit/vegetables

tuna, bean and apple salad

This tasty and refreshing salad is easily assembled from some fresh fruit and vegetables and pantry ingredients. It also makes a great filling for pita bread or topping for baked potatoes.

SERVES 4

2 x 14-ounce cans cannellini beans, drained	**For the dressing**
1 red onion, very thinly sliced	3 tablespoons extra virgin olive oil
2 red peppers, seeded and thinly sliced	2 teaspoons Dijon mustard
12 ounces mixed cherry tomatoes (red, yellow, orange), halved	3 teaspoons cider vinegar
	Zest of 1 clementine
2 tablespoons chopped fresh herbs (flat-leaf parsley, mint and chives)	Salt and freshly ground black pepper
2 x 7-ounce cans tuna in olive oil, drained	
2 dessert apples	

In a large serving bowl, combine the cannellini beans with the onion, peppers, tomatoes and herbs.

Break up the tuna into rough chunks and add to the bowl. Quarter the apples and remove the cores. Cut the quarters in half again and chop into thick slices before adding to the other ingredients.

Combine the dressing ingredients in a screw-top jar and shake well to mix. Pour over the salad and stir gently until all the ingredients are coated. Serve at once.

If you are not a fan of raw onion, try making this with the marinated onion from the Warm Chicken and Pink Grapefruit Salad recipe (page 75). An alternative dressing can be made from 2 tablespoons horseradish sauce combined with 2 tablespoons nonfat Greek yogurt.

Chosen as a source of: vitamins B6, B12, C, D, E, folate, selenium, MUFA, fish/seafood, pulses, polyphenols / Per serving: 422 kcal; 17.4g fat; 2.8g saturated fat / 4 portions of fruit/vegetables

crab and avocado salad

A simple salad but packed with flavor and beneficial nutrients. Makes a lovely summer lunch.

SERVES 4

½ large cucumber
2 medium ripe avocados
9 ounces crabmeat (fresh or canned)
3½ ounces watercress

For the dressing
2 tablespoons fish sauce
Zest and juice of 1 lime

2 teaspoons sesame oil
2 tablespoons palm sugar or golden superfine sugar
4 scallions, finely sliced
1 small red chili, seeded and finely chopped
A small handful of fresh flat-leaf parsley or cilantro, chopped

To make the dressing mix the fish sauce, lime zest and juice, sesame oil and sugar in a small bowl and stir until the sugar dissolves. Add the scallions, chili and cilantro or parsley and mix well.

For the salad, cut the cucumber in half lengthwise and remove the seeds with a teaspoon. Cut the flesh into small cubes and place in a salad bowl.

Cut the avocados in half, carefully remove the pits and scoop out the flesh neatly using a tablespoon. Dice the flesh and add to the cucumber.

Drain the crabmeat, if using canned, and add to the avocado and cucumber. Mix gently to combine.

Pour the dressing over and toss lightly. Serve on a bed of watercress with some crusty bread or toasted ciabatta.

Using cooked, peeled shrimp instead of the crabmeat also works well.

Chosen as a source of: vitamins B6, C, E, MUFA, fish/seafood / Per serving (not including bread): 281 kcal; 20g fat; 4.1g saturated fat / 2 portions of fruit/vegetables

roasted vegetable and mixed grain salad

You can serve this salad warm or cold and it makes a good light lunch or a substantial side dish. Roasting the vegetables gives them a lovely smoky flavor and, if you can find red quinoa, it will add further color and interest.

SERVES 4–6

2 medium sweet potatoes, peeled and cut into bite-size pieces
1 zucchini, cut into bite-size pieces
3 small shallots, quartered
2 tablespoons olive oil
2 garlic cloves, crushed or finely chopped
1 teaspoon cumin
3½ ounces (about ½ cup) quinoa

3½ ounces (about ½ cup) bulgur wheat
2 scallions, sliced on the diagonal
2 tablespoons finely chopped mint
2 large handfuls of arugula leaves, roughly chopped
Juice of 1 lime
1 tablespoon sunflower seeds

Preheat the oven to 350°F.

Place the sweet potato, zucchini and shallots on a baking sheet lined with parchment paper. Combine the olive oil, garlic and cumin and drizzle over the vegetables, ensuring they are all coated. Bake the vegetables for 20–25 minutes or until soft.

Meanwhile, follow the package instructions to cook the quinoa and bulgur wheat and drain.

Place the grains in a salad bowl, add the scallions, mint, arugula and lime juice and stir to combine. Gently stir in the roasted vegetables, taking care not to mash them.

Sprinkle the sunflower seeds over and serve.

Try roasting other vegetables such as pumpkin, peppers or beet.

Chosen as a source of: vitamins B6, C, folate, polyphenols / Per serving (based on serving 4): 365 kcal; 8.9g fat; 1.2g saturated fat / 2.5 portions of fruit/vegetables

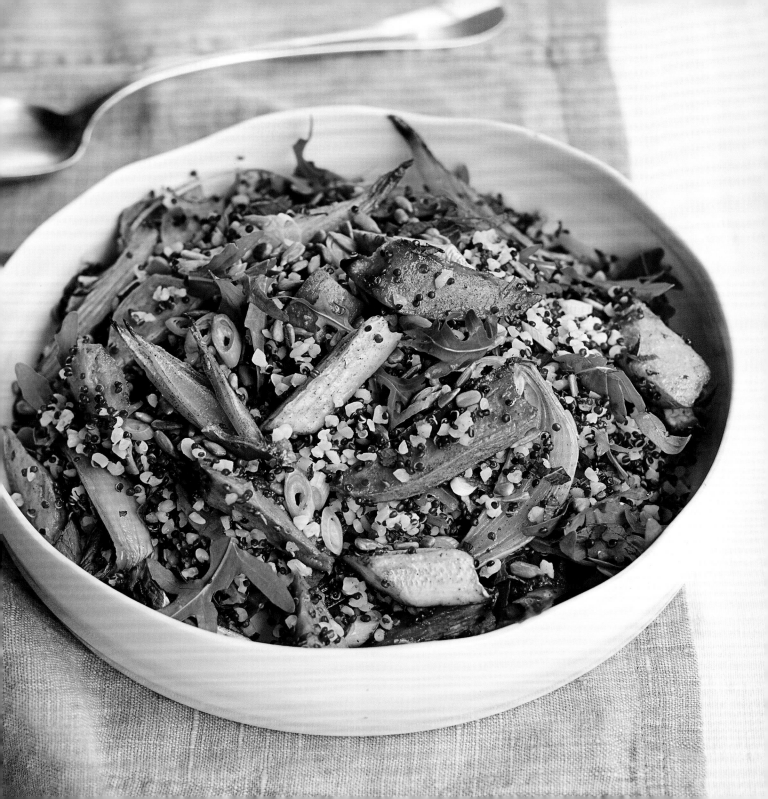

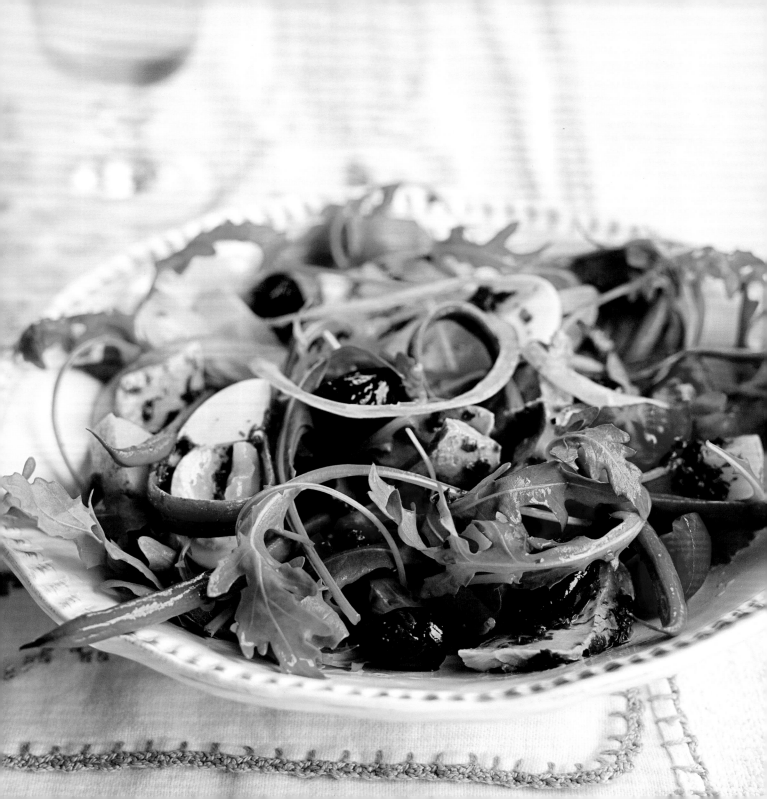

salad niçoise

A classic salad that is perfect for a light meal. We have used fresh tuna here to maximize the healthy long-chain omega-3 fatty acids (these are missing from canned tuna).

SERVES 4

2 free-range eggs
11¼ ounces baby new potatoes
3½ ounces French beans
10½ ounces tuna steaks
1 teaspoon olive oil
3½ ounces arugula leaves
16 cherry tomatoes, halved
1 small red onion, thinly sliced
¾ ounce canned anchovy fillets
   in oil, drained
A handful of black olives

Salt and freshly ground black
   pepper

For the dressing
½ small bunch of fresh basil
1 garlic clove
1 tablespoon fresh lemon juice
3 tablespoons olive oil
Salt and freshly ground black
   pepper

Preheat a griddle pan or broiler.

Boil the eggs in a pan of water for 10 minutes until hard-boiled. Drain and cool. Peel under cold water and quarter.

Meanwhile, cook the potatoes in boiling water for about 15–20 minutes or until tender, adding the beans for the last 5 minutes. Drain the potatoes and beans and run under cold water. Cut the potatoes into quarters.

Brush the tuna with the olive oil and season all over with salt and pepper. Cook the steaks for about 2 minutes on each side, either under the broiler or in a griddle pan. Remove from heat and flake or slice into strips.

Combine all the dressing ingredients using a food-processor or pestle and mortar.

In a serving bowl, toss together the potatoes, beans, arugula, tomatoes, onion and most of the dressing. Arrange the egg quarters and tuna on top, followed by the anchovies, then sprinkle with olives and drizzle with the remaining dressing.

Chosen as a source of: vitamins B6, B12, C, D, folate, selenium, MUFA, fish/seafood, pulses, polyphenols / Per serving: 328 kcal; 17.8g fat; 3.5g saturated fat / 1.5 portions of fruit/vegetables

smoked trout and lima bean salad

This is a very simple but really tasty salad that can be ready in just a few minutes.

SERVES 4

9 ounces hot smoked trout
   fillets, broken into large flakes
4 tomatoes, cut into small
   wedges
14-ounce can lima beans,
   drained
3½ ounces arugula leaves

For the dressing
1 slice lean back bacon,
   chopped
1 garlic clove, crushed
Scant ½ cup white wine
1 tablespoon finely chopped
   fresh flat-leaf parsley
1 tablespoon finely chopped
   fresh mint

In a large serving dish, combine the flaked trout, tomato wedges, lima beans and arugula.

To make the dressing, dry-fry the bacon in a nonstick pan until golden. Add the garlic and white wine and allow to bubble for 1–2 minutes for the flavors to combine.

Stir the parsley and mint into the bacon dressing then pour over the salad ingredients and combine gently.

The salad also works well using cold poached salmon or canned tuna, but remember that canned tuna is not a source of healthy, long-chain omega-3 fatty acids.

Chosen as a source of: vitamins B6, B12, C, D, E, folate, fish/seafood, pulses, polyphenols / Per serving: 205 kcal; 5.9g fat; 1.5g saturated fat / 2 portions of fruit/vegetables

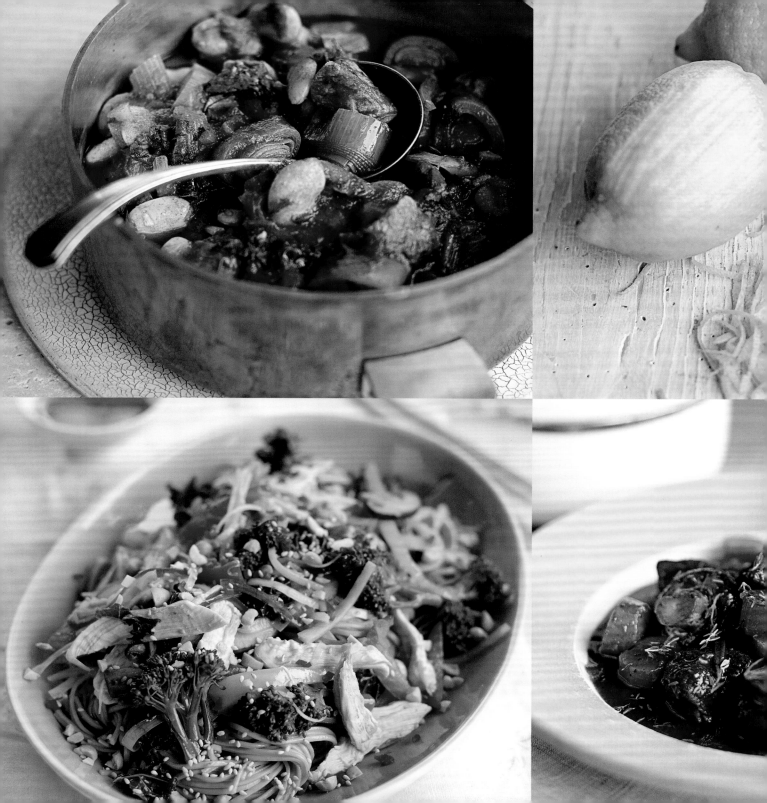

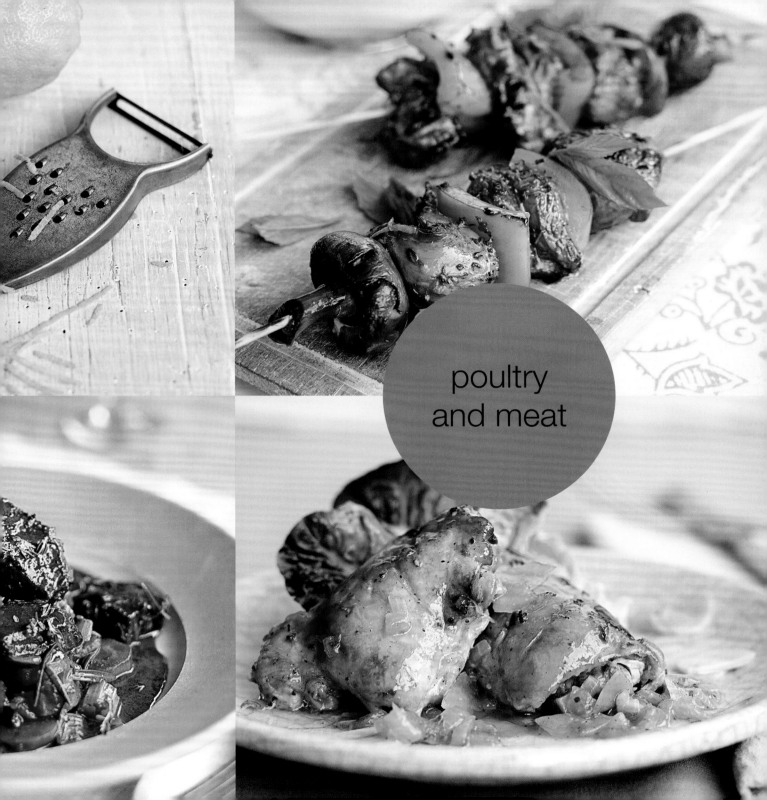

poultry
and meat

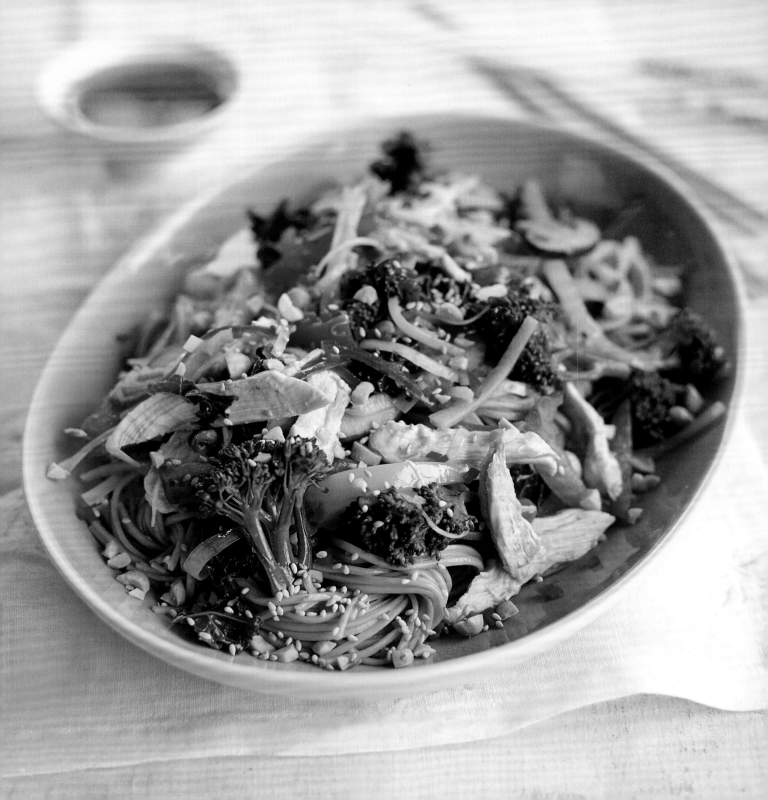

thai stir-fry with green tea noodles

A versatile recipe full of aromatic, zingy flavors.

SERVES 4

3½ ounces broccoli florets
1 tablespoon canola oil
1 red onion, very thinly sliced
1 leek, cleaned and shredded
2 carrots, cut into matchsticks
1 red and 1 yellow pepper,
   seeded and sliced
3½ ounces kale or cavalo nero,
   leaves only, shredded
2¾ ounces chestnut
   mushrooms, washed
   and sliced
9 ounces cooked turkey or
   chicken
2 tablespoons toasted sesame
   seeds (optional)

For the noodles
Zest and juice of 1 lime
1 teaspoon palm sugar
2 teaspoons fish sauce
1 teaspoon sesame oil
1 tablespoon sweet chili sauce
7 ounces green tea noodles
1 ounce chopped peanuts
½ red chili, seeded and very
   finely chopped (optional)

For the sauce
Zest and juice of 1 lime
1 teaspoon palm sugar
2 teaspoons fish sauce
1 teaspoon sesame oil
1 tablespoon sweet chili sauce

Blanch the broccoli florets in boiling water for 2 minutes. Drain.

To prepare the noodles, mix together the lime zest and juice, palm sugar, fish sauce, sesame oil and sweet chili sauce in a bowl. Cook the noodles according to the package instructions. Drain and add to the bowl along with the peanuts and chili, if using. Keep warm while you make the stir-fry.

Heat the canola oil in a wok over high heat. Once very hot, add the onion, leek and carrots and stir-fry for 2 minutes. Add the broccoli, peppers, kale and mushrooms and stir-fry for a further 2 minutes. Add the turkey or chicken and cook for 1 minute.

Mix the sauce ingredients together and pour into the wok. Once the sauce is bubbling, reduce the heat and toss gently to coat. Divide the noodles between four bowls, top with the stir-fry, sprinkle over the sesame seeds (if using) and serve.

Green tea noodles are available from Chinese or Asian supermarkets but soba or rice noodles work just as well.

Chosen as a source of: vitamins B6, C, E, folate, polyphenols / Per serving: 454 kcal; 13.8g fat; 2.3g saturated fat / 3.5 portions of fruit/vegetables

chicken satay with peanut sauce

These chicken kebabs are packed full of flavor.

SERVES 4

4 skinless chicken fillets, cut
   into bite-size cubes
1 green and 1 yellow pepper
12 cherry tomatoes

For the peanut sauce
3½ ounces dry-roasted peanuts
2 garlic cloves, roughly
   chopped
½ teaspoon reduced-salt soy
   sauce
2 tablespoons brown sugar
2 tablespoons fish sauce
½ teaspoon cayenne pepper
   or 1 fresh chili, chopped
5 tablespoons reduced-fat
   coconut milk
1 teaspoon sesame oil
½ tablespoon lime juice
5 tablespoons water

For the marinade
1 tablespoon lemon juice
1 tablespoon brown sugar
1 tablespoon olive oil
1 small onion, finely chopped
3 garlic cloves, crushed
2-inch piece of fresh ginger,
   peeled and grated
½ teaspoon ground turmeric
2 tablespoons ground coriander
1 teaspoon chili powder or
   1 fresh chili, finely chopped
3 tablespoons reduced-salt soy
   sauce
2 tablespoons fish sauce
1 tablespoon chopped and
   crushed lemongrass

8 skewers (if wooden, soak in
   water first)

Mix the marinade ingredients together in a shallow bowl. Add the chicken and stir well to coat. Cover and leave to marinate in the refrigerator for at least 12 hours.

For the peanut sauce, place all the ingredients in a blender or food-processor and process until smooth. Taste and adjust the flavoring if needed. Add a little more water if needed.

For the kebabs, thread the marinated chicken onto skewers, alternating with pieces of pepper and cherry tomatoes. Broil under a medium heat until the chicken is cooked through, turning and basting with the remaining marinade occasionally. Alternatively, grill on a barbecue.

Gently heat the peanut sauce in a pan over medium heat until warmed through. Serve the kebabs with the peanut dipping sauce and a large green salad.

Chosen as a source of: vitamins B6, C, folate, selenium, MUFA, pulses, polyphenols / Per serving: 458 kcal; 21g fat; 4.9g saturated fat / 0.5 portions of fruit/vegetables

moroccan-style chicken couscous

The apricots in this dish contrast beautifully with the intense Moroccan spices. It's worth trying to get hold of the spice mix ras el hanout as this imparts a unique flavor.

SERVES 4

5½ ounces (about 1 scant cup) couscous
¾ cup hot chicken stock
3 tablespoons canola oil
3 skinless chicken breasts, cut into bite-size pieces
1 red onion, thinly sliced
1 garlic clove, crushed or finely chopped
1 tablespoon ras el hanout (or 1 teaspoon cumin and 1 teaspoon ground coriander)

1 tablespoon tomato paste
14-ounce can chickpeas, drained
6–8 soft dried apricots, thinly sliced (pre-soak if needed)
A large handful of fresh cilantro, roughly chopped

Place the couscous in a serving bowl, pour over the stock, cover with plastic wrap and leave for 10 minutes.

Heat 1 tablespoon of the oil in a frying pan and cook the chicken on high heat until just browned but not cooked through, then remove from the pan and set aside.

Reduce the heat, add the remainder of the oil to pan and cook the onion and garlic until soft and translucent. Add the spices and cook for a further minute before stirring in the tomato paste.

Return the chicken to the pan and continue to cook for 2–3 minutes until the chicken is cooked through. Add the chickpeas and apricots and cook for a further minute to heat through.

Use a fork to fluff up the couscous. Add the chicken mix and the cilantro and stir to distribute evenly. Serve hot or cold.

Chosen as a source of: vitamins B6, E, folate, selenium, pulses, polyphenols / Per serving: 449 kcal; 13.7g fat; 1.3g saturated fat / 2 portions of fruit/vegetables

lemon chicken

Thank you to Dr. John Rayman for sharing this recipe; it has been a firm favorite in his repertoire for many years. The chicken needs to be marinated the day before for the best results, but after that it is as simple as popping into the oven.

SERVES 4

2 lemons
1 large onion, roughly chopped
2 garlic cloves, crushed or very thinly sliced
1 tablespoon honey

8 lean chicken thighs (about 14 ounces), skin and fat removed
Salt and freshly ground black pepper

Squeeze the juice from one of the lemons and set aside. Use a paring knife to remove the zest from the other lemon and cut it into pieces about ½-inch square. Remove any white pith from the skinned lemon, slice it thinly, and then chop the slices into coin-size pieces. Remove the pips and put the lemon pieces into a shallow baking dish. Add the onion, garlic and honey and season to taste with black pepper and salt, if required.

Use a sharp knife to cut a few deep slashes in each chicken thigh and then add the chicken to the dish. Use your hands to work the lemon and onion mixture into the chicken. Cover with plastic wrap and put in the refrigerator overnight.

Preheat the oven to 350°F.

Cook the chicken for 45–60 minutes, uncovered, turning the chicken pieces over from time to time so that they are browned on both sides. When the thighs are cooked, they should be flecked with charred points.

Serve with rice or potatoes and accompany with a green salad or the French Lentil Salad on page 76.

This would work equally well with the same weight of turkey thighs if you prefer.

Chosen as a source of: vitamins B6, B12, C, selenium, polyphenols / Per serving: 232 kcal; 8.9g fat; 2.5g saturated fat / 0.5 portions of fruit/vegetables

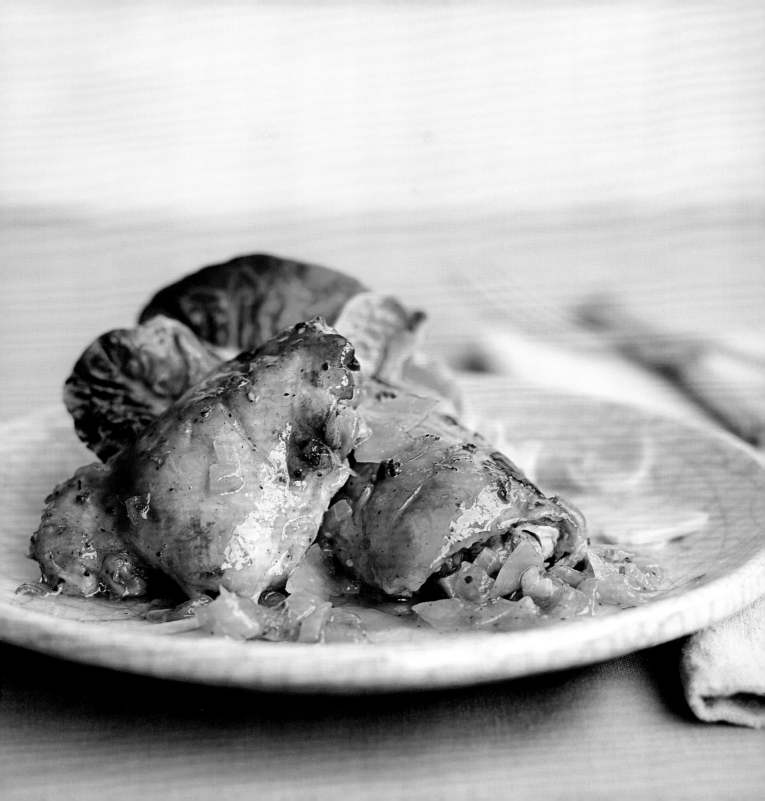

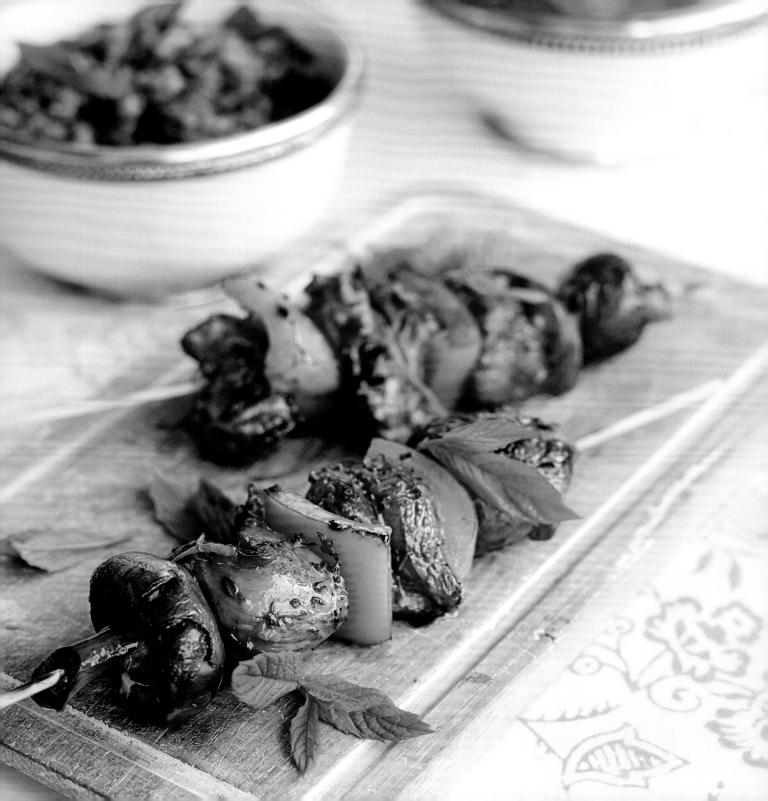

lamb souvlaki with warm lentil salad

A delicious variation on a traditional Greek recipe. The marinade ingredients are not wasted, as they are used to flavor the delicious lentils.

SERVES 6

2 pounds 4 ounces lean lamb leg meat, cubed

2 orange or red peppers, seeded and cut into large chunks

7 ounces chestnut mushrooms,

For the lentils

7 ounces (1¼ cups) large green lentils, washed and drained

1 echalion (banana) shallot, peeled and finely chopped

¾ ounce fresh mint, chopped

For the marinade

1½ tablespoons dried thyme

6 garlic cloves, crushed

Zest and juice of 3 lemons

3½ tablespoons olive oil

Scant ²/₃ cup red wine

½ teaspoon dried chili flakes

12 skewers (if wooden, soak in water first)

Mix together the marinade ingredients in a non-metallic bowl. Add the lamb, stir, cover and marinate for 3–4 hours or overnight in the refrigerator.

Remove the lamb from the marinade with a slotted spoon and thread onto skewers, alternating with chunks of pepper and whole mushrooms. Brush with some of the marinade.

Pour the remainder of the marinade into a measuring cup and top up to 1¾ cups with water. Pour into a medium pan with the lentils and shallot. Bring to a boil, then reduce the heat and simmer, covered, for 35–40 minutes until the lentils are just tender and the liquid has been absorbed.

Meanwhile, heat the broiler to high or use a griddle pan. Cook the kebabs in batches for 9–12 minutes, turning frequently, until the lamb is tender and the vegetables slightly charred.

Stir the mint through the lentils and pile onto a serving dish. Place the kebabs on top and serve with a bowl of green salad.

Chosen as a source of: vitamins B6, B12, C, folate, selenium, MUFA, pulses, polyphenols / Per serving: 475 kcal; 23g fat; 7.1g saturated fat / 1.5 portions of fruit/vegetables

lamb provençale

This delicious dish is bursting with the flavors of the Mediterranean. Thanks to Katie's mum, Pat Sanger, for sharing this recipe and for fond memories of eating this as a child.

SERVES 6

2¹/₃ tablespoons all-purpose flour

1 tablespoon canola oil

1 pound 10 ounces lean lamb leg meat, cubed

1 large onion, sliced

2 garlic cloves, crushed

1 green, 1 red and 1 yellow pepper, seeded and sliced

14-ounce can chopped tomatoes

2 tablespoons tomato paste

3½ cups beef or lamb stock

1¼ cups red wine

2 bay leaves

7 ounces mushrooms, thickly sliced

Salt and freshly ground black pepper

Preheat the oven to 350°F.

Place the flour in a large plastic bag, tip in the lamb cubes and shake until the meat is coated.

In a large flameproof casserole (cast-iron if you have one), heat the oil over medium heat until quite hot. Fry the lamb cubes until lightly browned on all sides. Remove with a slotted spoon and set aside. Turn the heat down to medium.

Add the onion and garlic to the pan (with a little more oil if needed) and cook for a few minutes until translucent. Return the lamb to the casserole along with all the other ingredients except the mushrooms.

Bring to a boil on top of the stove then cover and place in the oven to cook for about 1 hour. Remove from the oven and stir in the mushrooms. Reduce the temperature to 320°F and return the casserole to the oven for a further 30–40 minutes.

The lamb will be meltingly tender and the sauce rich and thick. Serve with green vegetables and potatoes or rice and a green salad.

Chosen as a source of: vitamins B6, B12, C, E, folate, polyphenols / Per serving: 379 kcal; 15.6g fat; 5.1g saturated fat / 2.5 portions of fruit/vegetables

liver, apple and bacon

This simple, one-pot meal is the perfect dish for those new to cooking or eating liver.

SERVES 4–6

1 pound 9 ounces tart apples, peeled, cored and thinly sliced
2 onions, thinly sliced
6 sage leaves
14 ounces calves' liver, cut into bite-size pieces
14-ounce can chopped tomatoes

4 slices lean back bacon, fat removed, chopped into bite-size pieces
Generous 1 cup beef stock
Salt and freshly ground black pepper

Preheat the oven to 350°F.

Put about one-third of the apple and onion slices on the bottom of a casserole dish. Scatter the sage leaves over the top.

Cover with half the liver, then half the tomatoes with their liquid, and a third of the bacon. Season with salt and pepper.

Repeat the layers, finishing with a layer of apple and onion slices. Pour in the stock and place the remaining bacon on top.

Cook the casserole, covered, for 1 hour, before uncovering and cooking for a further 30 minutes to crisp up the bacon. Serve with steamed green vegetables and crusty bread to soak up the wonderful sauce.

Lambs' liver could also be used for this dish.

Chosen as a source of: vitamins B6, B12, C, E, folate, selenium, polyphenols / Per serving (based on 4 servings): 285 kcal; 6.3g fat; 1.9g saturated fat / 3 portions of fruit/vegetables

warming pork and lima bean stew

A tasty family meal and a great way to incorporate some pulses into your diet.

SERVES 4

2 tablespoons canola oil
1 pound 5 ounces lean pork, diced
1 onion, diced
3 garlic cloves, crushed or finely chopped
2 sticks celery, thickly sliced
2 leeks, thickly sliced
1 teaspoon ground coriander
1 teaspoon ground cumin

1 tablespoon harissa paste
2 tablespoons tomato paste
14-ounce can chopped tomatoes
Generous 2 cups vegetable stock
14-ounce can lima beans, drained and rinsed
2 tablespoons roughly chopped cilantro

Preheat the oven to 350°F.

Add half the canola oil to a casserole dish and brown the cubed pork pieces over medium-high heat. Remove from the pan and set aside.

Add the remaining oil to the pan and fry the onion, garlic, celery and leeks over medium heat until slightly soft, about 3–4 minutes.

Return the pork to the pan and add the ground coriander, cumin, harissa paste and tomato paste and fry for a further 2 minutes. Add the chopped tomatoes and stock, bring to a boil and then transfer to the oven.

Cook for 50 minutes (or until the pork is tender). Check after 30 minutes and add more water if needed.

Add the lima beans and return to the oven for 5 minutes to heat through. Stir in the fresh cilantro and serve.

Chosen as a source of: vitamins B6, B12, C, E, folate, selenium, pulses, polyphenols / Per serving: 383 kcal; 14.1g fat; 2.7g saturated fat / 4 portions of fruit/vegetables

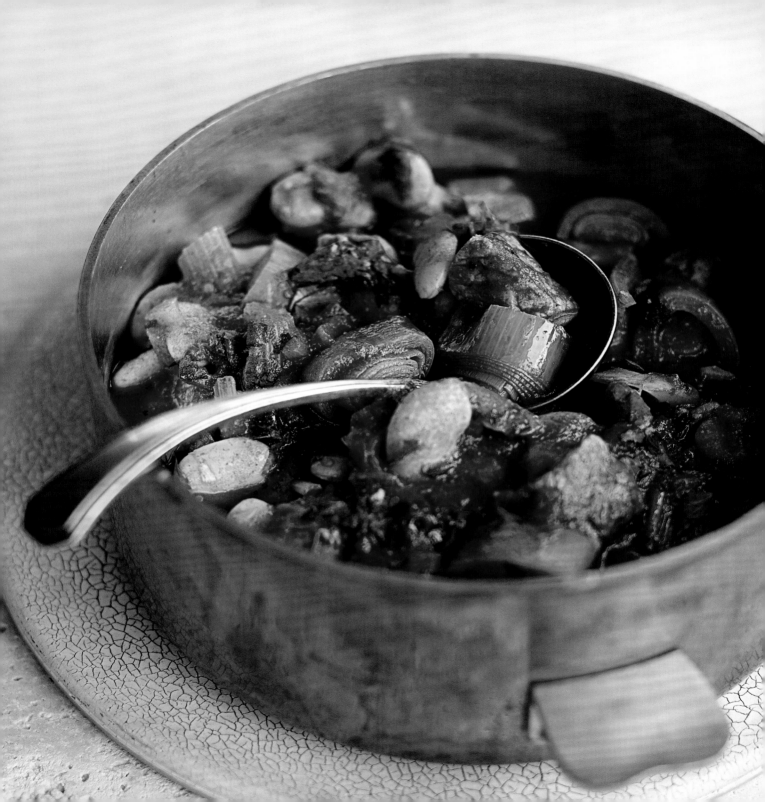

moroccan-spiced slow-cooked beef

Despite the three-hour cooking time, this is a really easy meal to prepare and gives melt-in-the-mouth tender beef. Ideally serve with couscous or some crusty bread.

SERVES 4

1¾ pounds lean beef, cubed into bite-size pieces
2 small onions, finely chopped
4 garlic cloves, crushed or finely chopped
2 teaspoons ras el hanout (or 1 teaspoon cumin and 1 teaspoon coriander)
½ teaspoon harissa paste or 1 teaspoon paprika
½ teaspoon salt and pepper
14-ounce can chopped tomatoes
Juice of 1 and finely sliced zest of ½ lemon
2 teaspoons honey
3 tablespoons freshly chopped cilantro
2 tablespoons freshly chopped flat-leaf parsley

Preheat the oven to 300°F.

Set aside 2 tablespoons of the chopped cilantro for serving.

Place all the other ingredients in a casserole dish, add a scant ½ cup of water and stir to combine.

Place in the oven and cook for 3 hours. Check three-quarters of the way through the cooking time and add a little more water if needed.

Sprinkle with remaining cilantro before serving.

Chosen as a source of: vitamins B6, B12, C, folate, polyphenols / Per serving: 325 kcal; 11.9g fat; 4.8g saturated fat / 1.5 portions of fruit/vegetables

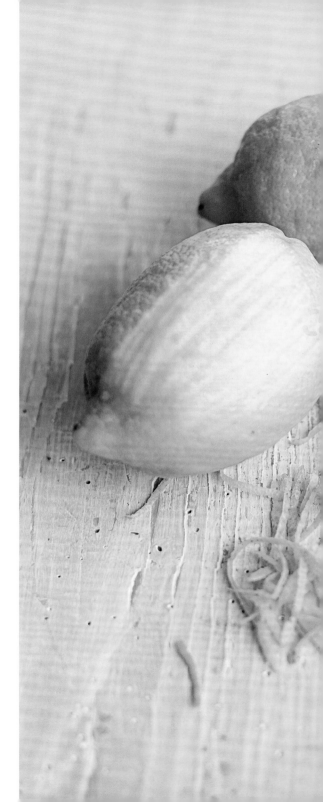

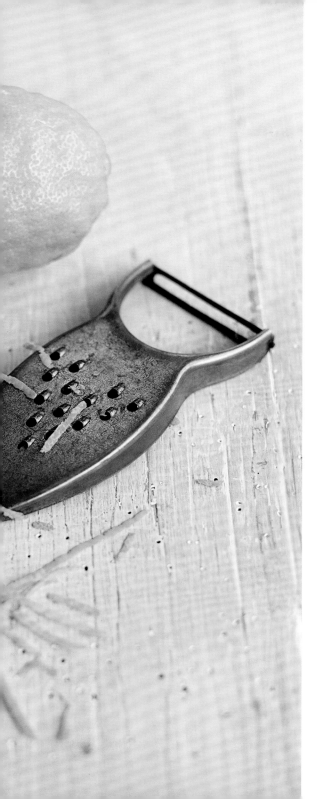

lemon and herb meatballs

This is great served with fresh wholegrain bread to soak up the sauce, which is packed with flavor.

SERVES 4

For the meatballs
1 small onion, roughly chopped
4 tablespoons freshly chopped flat-leaf parsley
A large handful of spinach (about 1¾ ounces), roughly chopped
14 ounces lean ground beef
1 free-range egg
2 slices wholewheat bread, broken into crumbs
½ teaspoon ground cumin
½ teaspoon paprika
½ teaspoon freshly ground black pepper
½ teaspoon salt
1 tablespoon olive oil
Zest of ½ and juice of 1 lemon

For the sauce
1 small onion, finely chopped
½ teaspoon paprika
½ teaspoon turmeric
¼ teaspoon ground cumin
1 red chili, finely chopped (or ½ teaspoon chili flakes)
1¾ cups hot vegetable stock
2 tablespoons freshly chopped cilantro

To make the meatballs, put the onion, half the parsley and the spinach in a food-processor and process until finely chopped.

In a separate bowl, mix together the ground beef, egg, breadcrumbs, cumin, paprika and salt and pepper. Add the processed onion, parsley and spinach to the bowl and knead well to form a paste-like consistency. Shape the mixture into walnut-size balls.

Heat the oil in a casserole or large, deep-sided frying pan with a lid. Brown the meatballs in batches and set aside.

To make the sauce, add the onion to the casserole and cook over gentle heat until soft. Add a little more olive oil if needed. Add the paprika, turmeric, cumin and chili and cook for a further minute. Add the stock and cilantro and bring to a boil.

Add the meatballs to the sauce, cover and simmer for 45 minutes. Add 1 tablespoon of the remaining parsley, the lemon juice and zest and simmer for another 2 minutes. Serve sprinkled with the remaining parsley.

Chosen as a source of: vitamins B6, B12, C, folate, MUFA, polyphenols / Per serving: 297 kcal; 15.3g fat; 5.2g saturated fat / 0.5 portions of fruit/ vegetables

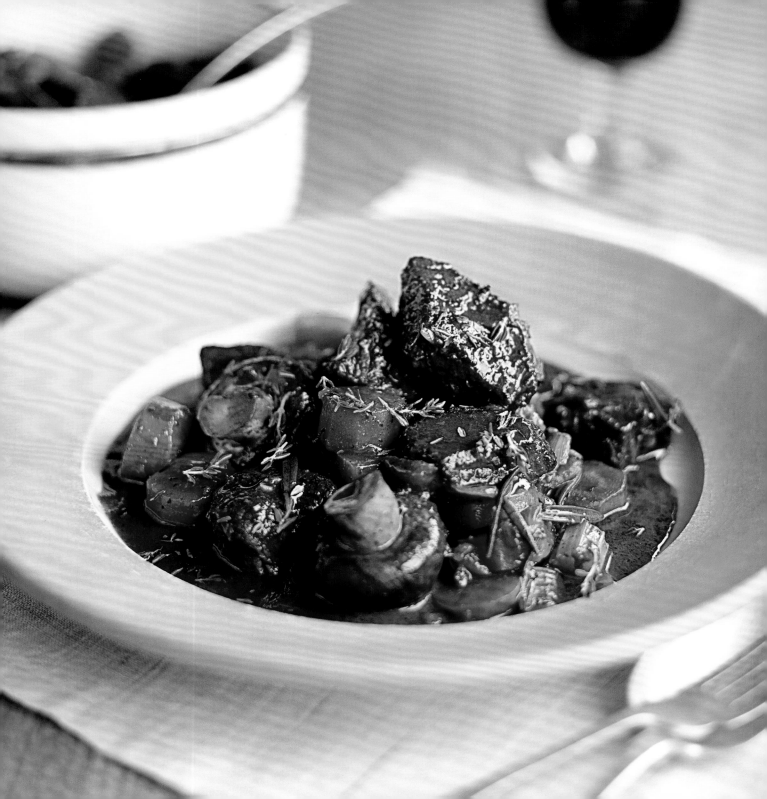

venison and chocolate casserole

Thank you to Dr. John Rayman for providing this beautifully rich and indulgent recipe.

SERVES 4

½ tablespoon olive oil (or use oil spray), plus extra as needed
5½ ounces lean smoked back bacon, diced
1 pound 9 ounces diced venison leg
2–3 tablespoons all-purpose flour
3 garlic cloves
3 red onions, chopped
3 sticks celery, sliced
5 carrots, chopped
9 ounces mushrooms, quartered
1 tablespoon fresh or dried rosemary
1 tablespoon fresh or dried thyme
2 bay leaves
1½ cups red wine
Generous 1 cup beef stock
2 tablespoons redcurrant jelly
1¼ ounces bittersweet chocolate (minimum 70 percent cocoa solids), grated
Salt and freshly ground black pepper

Preheat the oven to 325°F.

Heat the oil or spray in a flameproof casserole dish and fry the bacon until browned. Remove from the pan and set aside in a warm place.

Dredge the venison in seasoned flour until coated and shake off any excess. Add a little more oil or spray to the casserole as necessary and then seal the venison, in batches, over medium-high heat. Remove from the pan and keep warm.

Add some more oil to the casserole if needed and fry the garlic, onions, celery, carrots and mushrooms gently until browned. Add the herbs and bay leaves and then return the venison and the bacon to the pan.

Add the red wine and stock, season with salt and pepper, and bring to a boil. Cover and cook in the oven until the meat is tender—about 1½ hours.

Remove the meat and vegetables from the casserole and keep warm. Bring the liquid to a boil and whisk in the redcurrant jelly. Taste and adjust the seasoning. Now slowly stir in the chocolate, whisking continuously. Return the meat and vegetables to the casserole and heat through. Serve with a green vegetable and potatoes.

Chosen as a source of: vitamins B6, C, folate, selenium, polyphenols / Per serving: 474 kcal; 12.3g fat; 5.3g saturated fat / 3 portions of fruit/ vegetables

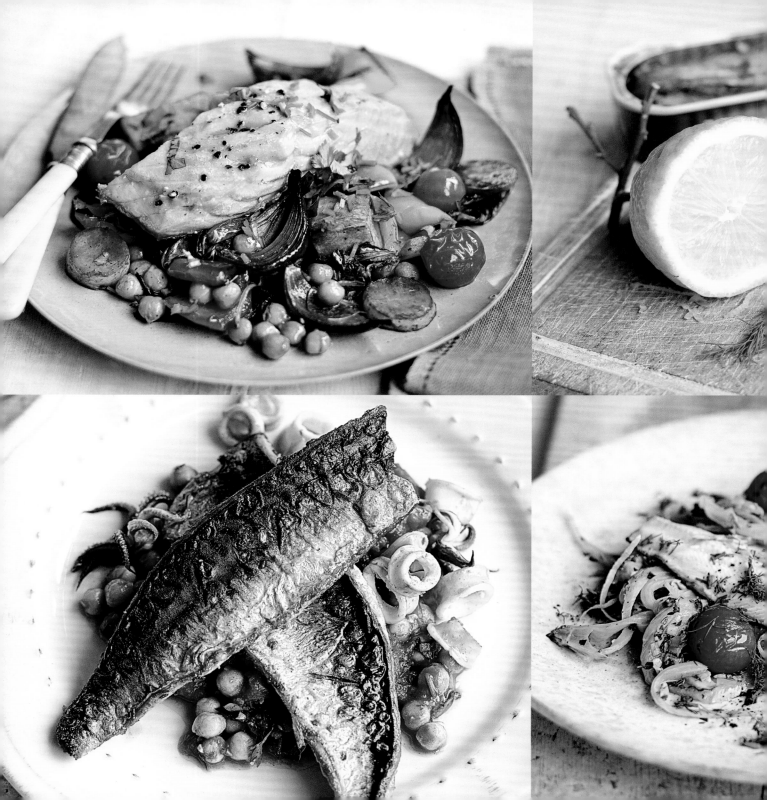

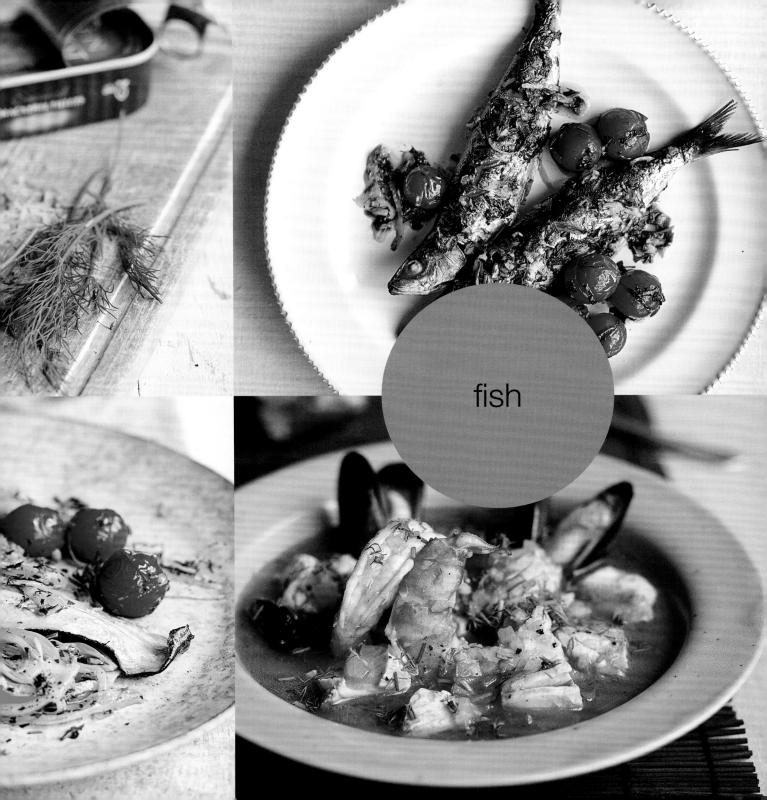

fish

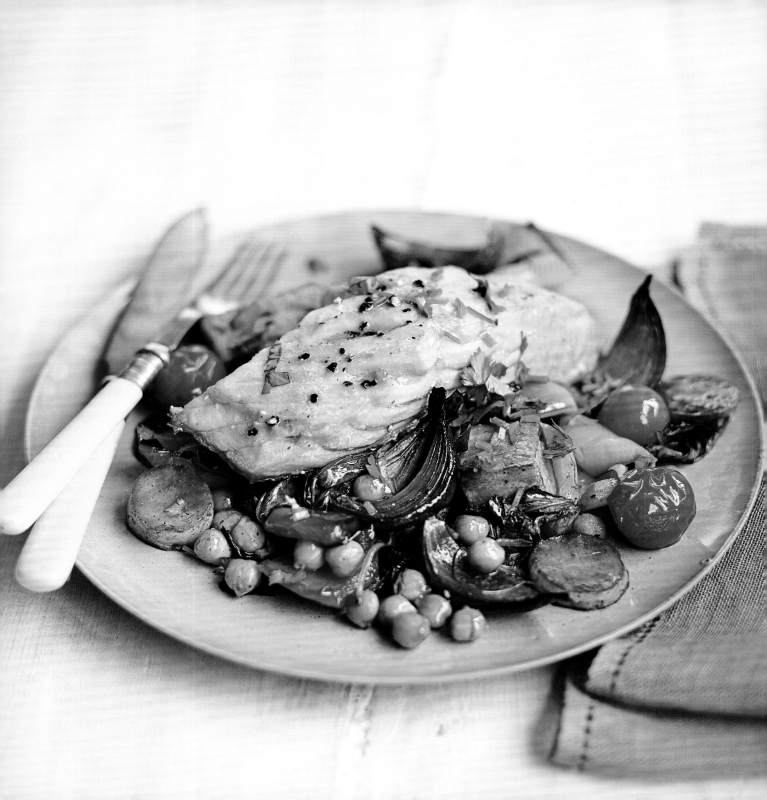

baked salmon with roasted vegetables

Whether you're cooking for a family supper or a smart dinner party, this quick and easy one-pot meal is perfect.

SERVES 4

2 medium sweet potatoes, peeled and cubed
1 red onion, cut into wedges
9 ounces cherry tomatoes
1 red and 1 yellow pepper, seeded and chopped
8 baby potatoes (about 10 ounces), washed and thinly sliced
2 tablespoons teriyaki sauce
2 tablespoons olive oil

½ x 14-ounce can chickpeas, rinsed and drained (about 4 ounces)
4 salmon fillets (each about 5½ ounces)
A large handful of spinach, washed and any tough stalks removed
A handful of cilantro, roughly chopped
Salt and freshly ground black pepper

Preheat the oven to 400°F.

Tip the sweet potatoes into a large, shallow roasting pan and add the onion, tomatoes, peppers and potatoes. Drizzle with 1 tablespoon of the teriyaki sauce and 1 tablespoon of the olive oil. Season with salt and pepper and toss everything together then spread out in an even layer in the pan. Roast for 30 minutes.

Stir in the chickpeas and top with the salmon. Season again and drizzle with the remaining teriyaki and olive oil. Roast for another 12 minutes until the salmon is just cooked and the vegetables tender.

Remove the salmon gently and set aside. Stir the spinach into the vegetable base. Serve the salmon on the bed of vegetables, scattered with cilantro.

Almost any type of vegetable can be used. Try pumpkin, marrows or mushrooms, or try increasing the amount of potatoes relative to sweet potatoes.

Chosen as a source of: vitamins B6, B12, C, D, E, folate, selenium, MUFA, fish/seafood, pulses, polyphenols / Per serving: 561 kcal; 25g fat; 4.2g saturated fat / 4 portions of fruit/vegetables

salmon with ginger and honey

The salmon in this recipe is cooked in a package of foil, which keeps it moist. This means you can prepare the packages a few hours ahead of time, pop them in the refrigerator, and then cook in the oven when needed. One big package or two individual ones can be used.

SERVES 2

Oil spray
2 salmon fillets (each about 5½ ounces)
1-inch piece of fresh ginger, peeled and thinly sliced

2 scallions, thinly sliced
1 tablespoon reduced-salt soy sauce
1 teaspoon honey
1 teaspoon sesame seeds (optional)

Preheat the oven to 350°F.

Lay out two pieces of foil—each one should be big enough to form a package around a salmon fillet. Grease each piece of foil with a spray or two of oil spray. Place a fillet in the center of each piece of foil.

Place equal amounts of the ginger and scallion on top of each fillet. Mix the soy sauce and the honey in a small bowl and pour over the fillets. Scatter with sesame seeds (if using).

Close up the packages loosely and cook in the preheated oven for 15 minutes. The fish is cooked when the flesh just flakes.

You could use sweet chili sauce instead of the honey or you could replace both soy sauce and honey with a tablespoon of teriyaki sauce.

Chosen as a source of: vitamins B6, B12, D, E, selenium, MUFA, fish/seafood / Per serving: 299 kcal; 17.7g fat; 3.1g saturated fat / 0 portions of fruit/vegetables

hearty fish pie

This pie is full of flavor and texture and looks really pretty. Most supermarkets now stock a fresh or frozen combination of fish suitable for pie filling.

SERVES 4

12 ounces sweet potatoes (about 2 medium), peeled and chopped
1 teaspoon dried dill
1 tablespoon olive oil
5¾ ounces broccoli florets
9¼ ounces fish-pie mix (salmon, cod, smoked haddock)
1½ cups skim milk
6 ounces cooked shrimp, drained if necessary
2 tablespoons chopped fresh dill
5 tablespoons cornstarch
1 pound 2 ounces cooked mashed potato
Salt and freshly ground black pepper

Preheat the oven to 375°F.

Toss the sweet potatoes with the dried dill and olive oil, spread in a single layer on a baking sheet and cook in the oven for 20 minutes until tender. Remove from the oven and set aside. Reduce the oven temperature to 350°F.

Meanwhile, blanch the broccoli in boiling water for 2 minutes, then drain. Poach the fish pieces in the milk for 3–5 minutes until just tender. Remove with a slotted spoon and place in the base of a large baking dish. Arrange the broccoli on top and then place the shrimp on top of the broccoli.

Add the fresh dill to the poaching liquid. In a bowl, add a couple of tablespoons of cold water to the cornstarch and mix to a paste. Add a ladleful of the warm poaching liquid to the paste and stir well. Transfer the loosened paste to the poaching pan and gradually bring to a boil, stirring continuously until the sauce thickens and begins to bubble. Taste and season, then pour the sauce over the fish, broccoli and shrimp.

Roughly mix the mashed potato with the roasted sweet potato so you can still see the sweet potato chunks and spread it evenly over the fish base. Rough up the top with a fork and then bake the pie in the oven for about 25 minutes until golden and crisp on top.

Chosen as a source of: vitamins B6, B12, C, E, folate, selenium, fish/seafood, polyphenols / Per serving: 390 kcal; 7g fat; 1.4g saturated fat / 2 portions of fruit/vegetables

spiced mackerel with smoky chickpeas

The strong flavor of mackerel works well with spice.

SERVES 4

4–6 mackerel fillets (about 1¾ pounds total), skin on and pin-boned
1 teaspoon each cumin and coriander seeds, toasted and crushed
½ teaspoon ground turmeric
½ teaspoon chili flakes
1 tablespoon olive oil
3–4 baby squid, cleaned and cut into rings (optional)

For the smoky chickpeas
1 tablespoon canola oil
1 echalion (banana) shallot, finely chopped
1–2 garlic cloves, finely chopped
1 teaspoon ground cumin
1 teaspoon smoked paprika
3½ tablespoons white wine or hard cider
Zest and juice of 1 lemon
Scant 1 cup vegetable stock
8-ounce can chopped tomatoes
14-ounce can chickpeas, drained
¾ ounce flat-leaf parsley, chopped

Make several slashes in the skin of each mackerel fillet with a sharp knife. Mix together the crushed seeds, turmeric, chili flakes and olive oil to make a paste and rub into the skin of each fillet. Set aside to marinate while you prepare the chickpeas.

Heat half of the canola oil in a large pan over medium heat. Add the shallot and cook gently for 5 minutes until softened. Add the garlic, cumin and paprika and cook for a further 2 minutes, adding a little water if needed. Add the wine or cider and lemon zest to the pan, stir well, and allow to bubble for a minute or two. Stir in the stock, tomatoes and chickpeas, and simmer gently, uncovered, for 20 minutes.

10 minutes before the chickpeas are ready, heat the remaining canola oil in a large nonstick frying pan until very hot. Place the mackerel fillets in the pan, skin-side down and cook without moving for 3 minutes until the skin is crispy. Turn the fillets over carefully, reduce the heat and cook for a further 2–3 minutes. Remove with a slotted spoon and keep warm. Add the squid to the hot pan and stir-fry for 2–3 minutes until opaque.

Stir the lemon juice and parsley into the chickpeas, divide between serving plates and top with the mackerel and squid.

Chosen as a source of: vitamins B6, B12, C, D, E, folate, selenium, MUFA, fish/seafood, pulses, polyphenols / Per serving: 609 kcal; 41g fat; 7.3g saturated fat / 1.5 portions of fruit/vegetables

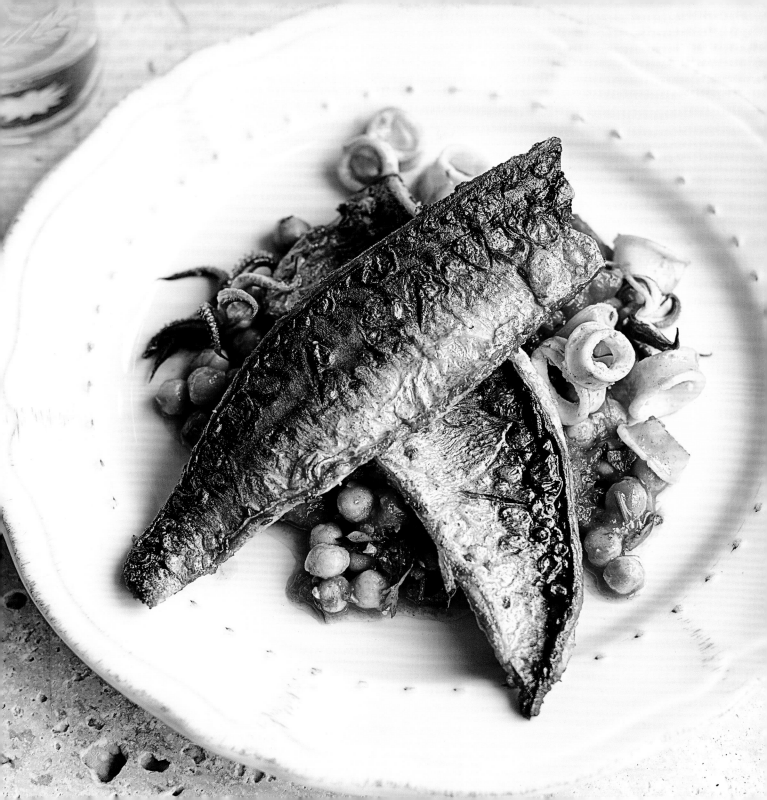

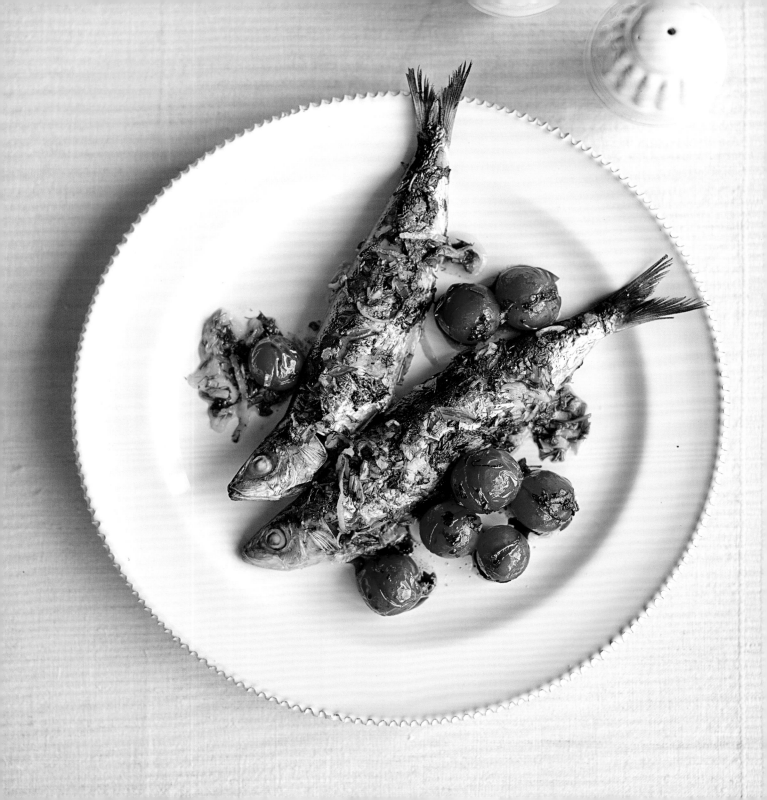

broiled sardines with balsamic roasted tomatoes

When available, fresh sardines make a very tasty meal. Here they are paired with lemon, garlic and herbs and served with roasted baby tomatoes.

SERVES 2

4–6 sardines, gutted and
  descaled

For the marinade
1 tablespoon olive oil
2 garlic cloves, crushed or finely
  chopped
Zest and juice of 1 lemon
1 tablespoon finely chopped dill
1 tablespoon finely chopped
  flat-leaf parsley

For the tomatoes
7 ounces cherry tomatoes
½ tablespoon olive oil
2 tablespoons balsamic vinegar
½ teaspoon dried oregano
1 tablespoon roughly chopped
  basil

Preheat the oven to 350°F.

Wash the sardines, removing the heads and tails if preferred, and pat dry with paper towels. Use a sharp knife to score a few cuts on each side of the sardines.

Make the marinade by combining the olive oil, garlic, lemon zest and juice with the dill and parsley in a small bowl. Rub the marinade all over the fish and into the cuts in the skin. Place any remaining marinade inside the fish and set aside while you prepare the tomatoes.

Place the tomatoes on a baking sheet. Add the olive oil, balsamic vinegar and herbs and coat well. Bake the tomatoes for approximately 20 minutes or until soft and glazed.

Broil the fish for about 2–4 minutes on each side until the skin is crisp and the flesh firm. Serve with the roasted tomatoes.

Chosen as a source of: vitamins B6, B12, C, D, E, folate, selenium, omega-3, MUFA, fish/seafood, polyphenols / Per serving: 283 kcal; 18.9g fat; 4.1g saturated fat / 1 portion of fruit/vegetables

sea bream provençale

Sea bream stands up well to the rich Provençale flavors and the skin stays nice and crispy.

SERVES 4

1 tablespoon olive oil, plus
  extra for greasing
1 large eggplant, trimmed and
  cut into ½-inch slices
1 tablespoon garlic-infused
  olive oil
1 red and 1 yellow pepper,
  seeded and thickly sliced
1 quantity of Tasty Tomato
  Sauce (page 145)

1 teaspoon dried mixed herbs
  or a handful of fresh chopped
  herbs such as thyme,
  oregano, rosemary
9 ounces spinach leaves
1 tablespoon canola oil
4 sea bream fillets (each about
  4½ ounces)

Preheat the oven to 350°F and grease a shallow baking dish with a little olive oil.

Brush the eggplant slices with the garlic-infused oil, place on a lined baking sheet and bake for 10 minutes. Toss the sliced peppers in the tablespoon of olive oil, add to the baking sheet with the eggplant, and bake for a further 10–15 minutes.

Mix the fresh or dried herbs with the tomato sauce and spread half the mixture in the base of the prepared dish. Arrange the eggplant slices in a layer on top of the sauce and scatter the peppers evenly on top of them. Cover with the remaining tomato sauce, then cover with foil and bake for 10 minutes. Remove the dish from the oven, scatter the spinach leaves on top, re-cover and return to the oven for a further 5 minutes.

Meanwhile, heat the canola oil in a large frying pan until very hot. Fry the fish fillets, skin side down, for 2–3 minutes until the skin is crisp and golden.

Remove the foil from the vegetables and gently stir the wilted spinach into the sauce. Place the sea bream fillets on top of the vegetables with the crispy skin uppermost. Return to the oven, uncovered, for a further 6–8 minutes until the fish is cooked through. Serve with crusty bread and a green salad or baked potatoes and a green vegetable.

Chosen as a source of: vitamins B6, B12, C, E, folate, MUFA, fish/seafood, polyphenols / Per serving: 282 kcal; 15.2g fat; 1.3g saturated fat / 3.5 portions of fruit/vegetables

trio of fishcakes

This selection of fishcakes is really tasty, quick and easy. The mackerel and sardine varieties are an ideal way to include more oily fish in your diet with minimal effort and maximum taste.

EACH RECIPE MAKES 4 SMALL FISHCAKES

Mackerel and Dill
9 ounces mashed potato
4½ ounced canned mackerel, drained
2 tablespoons chopped fresh dill or 1 teaspoon dried dill
Zest of 1 lemon

Sardine and Olive
9 ounces mashed potato
4¾ ounces canned sardines in olive oil with herbs, drained
¾ ounce snipped chives
½ teaspoon finely chopped fresh rosemary
½ ounce (2 tablespoons) pitted black olives, chopped

Tuna and Tomato
9 ounces mashed potato
7 ounces canned tuna in olive oil, drained
1½ ounces sun-dried tomatoes in olive oil, drained and chopped
1 ounce raw or marinated red onion (see Warm Chicken and Pink Grapefruit Salad, page 74), chopped

To finish (all recipes)
1 tablespoon all-purpose flour
1 free-range egg, lightly beaten
2 tablespoons fine cornmeal
Canola oil, for frying

The method for all three fishcakes is the same: flake the fish and mix loosely with the other ingredients. Chunks of fish should still be visible, so don't mash together too much. With damp hands, shape into four patties of equal size.

Have the flour, beaten egg and cornmeal ready in separate small dishes and dip the patties into each of these in turn so they have a thin coating of cornmeal on the outside.

For best results, fry in a little canola oil over medium heat for 4–5 minutes each side and drain on paper towels. The fishcakes can also be oven baked for about 20 minutes at 350ºF. They taste equally good but the texture is a little drier.

The fishcakes can be cooked without the flour-egg-cornmeal coating but will have a much softer texture.

Chosen as a source of: vitamins B6, B12, D, folate, selenium, fish/ seafood / Per fishcake (Mackerel and Dill): 216 kcal; 10.8g fat; 2.1g saturated fat / (Sardine and Olive): 202 kcal; 9g fat; 1.5g saturated fat / (Tuna and Tomato): 257 kcal; 10.2g fat; 1.8g saturated fat / 0.5 portions of fruit/vegetables

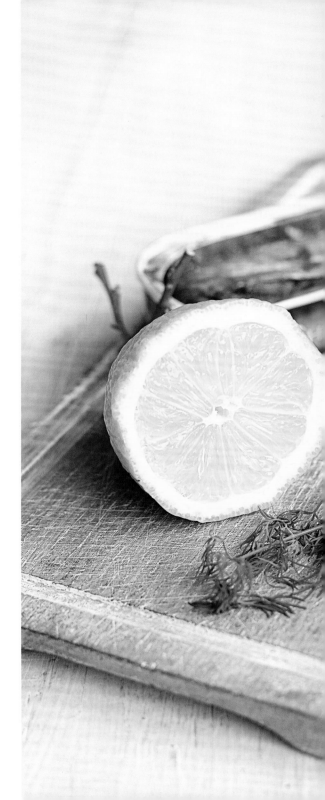

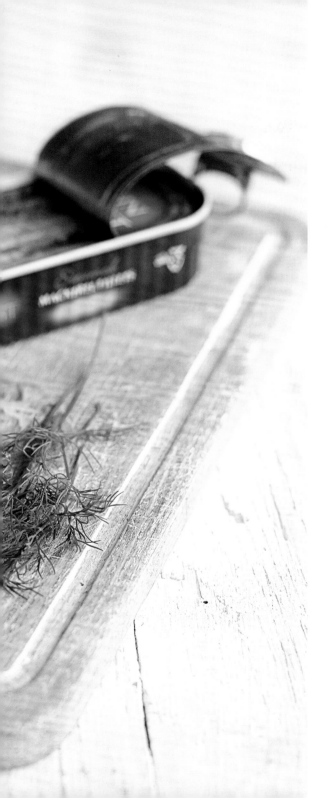

tapenade-topped cod

The tapenade on page 145 imparts a rich Mediterranean flavor to this tasty cod dish.

SERVES 4

4 cod fillets (about 5½ ounces each)
4–8 teaspoons tapenade (depending on taste)

2 tomatoes, sliced
1 lemon, sliced with the peel on
Salt and freshly ground black pepper

Preheat the oven to 400°F.

Place the cod on a baking sheet and spread 1–2 teaspoons of tapenade over each fillet. Arrange alternate slices of tomato and lemon on top of the tapenade.

Bake for 10–12 minutes until the fish is cooked through and opaque. Serve with some mixed salad leaves.

Any type of firm white fish could be used.

Chosen as a source of: vitamins B6, B12, C, selenium, fish/seafood, polyphenols / Per serving: 180 kcal; 5.9g fat; 0.8g saturated fat / 1 portion of fruit/vegetables

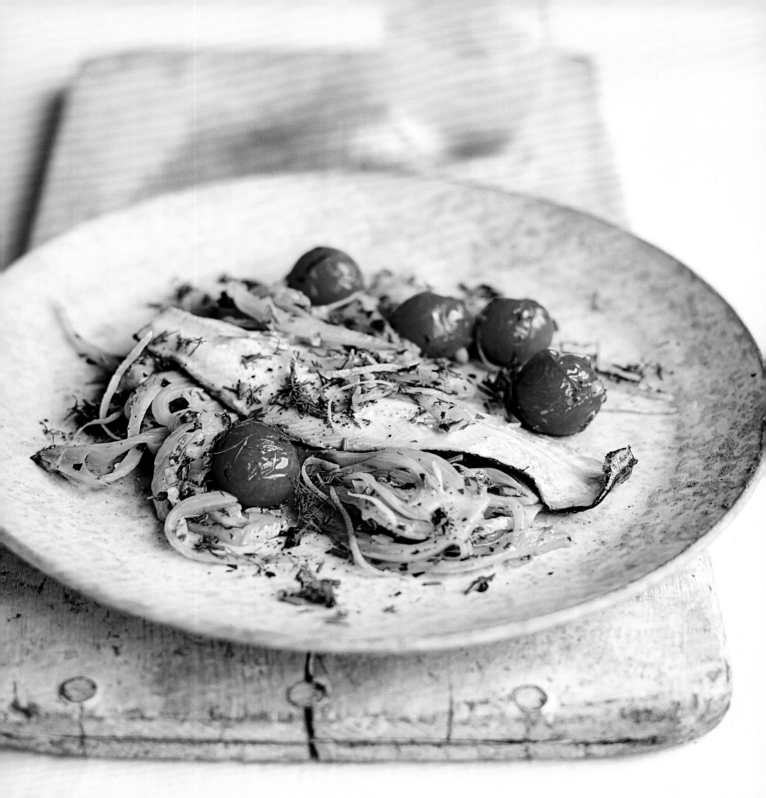

baked trout with white wine and fennel

This dish is so pretty it's almost a shame to eat it, but the flavors are fabulous. A real crowd-pleaser.

SERVES 4

Olive oil, for greasing
2 large or 3 smaller fennel bulbs, trimmed and thinly sliced
2 echalion (banana) shallots, finely chopped
2 garlic cloves, finely chopped
½ ounce fresh thyme leaves, chopped, or 1 teaspoon dried thyme
¾ ounce fresh flat-leaf parsley, chopped
Scant 1 cup dry white wine
4 trout fillets
Zest and juice of 1 lemon
10½ ounces cherry tomatoes
Chopped dill, to garnish
Salt and freshly ground black pepper

Preheat the oven to 400°F and grease a shallow baking dish with a little olive oil. A lasagna dish has good dimensions for this recipe.

Place the fennel, shallots, garlic, herbs and wine in the dish, stir, and season with pepper and a little salt. Cover the dish with a cartouche—a sheet of greased parchment paper that has been held under cold water and then squeezed to rid it of excess moisture. The paper should completely cover the fennel and be tucked inside the dish at the edges.

Cook in the oven for 25 minutes, stirring halfway through. Remove the paper and cook for a further 5–10 minutes. The fennel should be just tender and the aromas will be wonderful.

Reduce the oven temperature to 350°F. Place the trout fillets side by side on top of the fennel, squeeze over the lemon juice and arrange cherry tomatoes between the fillets and round the edge of the dish. Return to the oven and cook uncovered for 12–15 minutes, or until the trout is opaque and flakes easily.

Remove from the oven, garnish with lemon zest and dill and serve immediately with broccoli and sweet potato wedges.

Chosen as a source of: vitamins B6, B12, C, D, E, folate, selenium, fish/seafood, polyphenols / Per serving: 221 kcal; 6.8g fat; 1.4g saturated fat / 2.5 portions of fruit/vegetables

st clement's sole

The delicious sweet, sharp citrus flavors in this dish complement the sole beautifully and give the fish a lovely melt-in-the-mouth texture. This recipe is so easy and tasty that it's sure to become a great favorite.

SERVES 4

6 lemon sole fillets
Zest and juice of 1 lemon
Zest and juice of 1 lime
Zest and juice of 1 large orange
3 tablespoons dry white wine
2 tablespoons olive oil
¾ ounce fresh flat-leaf parsley, chopped
1 echalion (banana) shallot, finely chopped
Salt and freshly ground black pepper

Cut the sole fillets in half widthwise and arrange in a shallow baking dish.

Mix together the rest of the ingredients, season with black pepper and a little salt if required and pour evenly over the fish. Cover and leave to marinate for 30 minutes to 1 hour.

Preheat the oven to 400°F. When the fish has soaked up the citrus flavors, cover the dish tightly with foil and bake in the oven for 10–15 minutes until the fish is piping hot and flakes easily. Do not overcook—the citrus juices will have partially cooked the sole.

Serve straight from the dish with the delicious juices spooned on top. A good accompaniment is the French Lentil Salad on page 76 or plenty of green vegetables and some crushed new potatoes.

The marinade and cooking method would work well with most white fish but remember to adjust the cooking time according to the thickness of the fillets.

Chosen as a source of: vitamins, B12, C, folate, selenium, fish/seafood, polyphenols / Per serving: 216 kcal; 9.9g fat; 1.4g saturated fat / 0.5 portions of fruit/vegetables

salmon sushi rolls

With a bit of practice, sushi is actually quite easy to make and a great way to bring out the artist in you. We have kept the filling simple here with salmon and vegetables, but you can let your imagination run wild.

MAKES 24 BITE-SIZE ROLLS

2 sheets of nori seaweed, cut in half
2 ounces smoked salmon (or any sushi-grade raw fish), sliced into strips
6-inch piece of cucumber, peeled (optional) and cut into very thin batons
1 small carrot, cut into very fine batons

Wasabi paste (optional)
Reduced-salt soy sauce or teriyaki sauce, for dipping

For the rice
2 tablespoons rice vinegar
½ teaspoon sugar
¼ teaspoon salt
4½ ounces (about ⅔ cup) sushi rice

To prepare the rice, place the vinegar in a small bowl and stir in the sugar and salt until dissolved. Set aside.

Wash the rice well in cold water at least three times to remove excess starch. Drain well. Bring ⅔ cup of water to boil in a pan and add the rice. Simmer for 10 minutes with the lid on. Turn off the heat and leave to stand for a further 20 minutes with the lid on.

Place the rice in a non-metallic bowl. Add the vinegar mixture and gently cut it in with a wooden spatula, being careful not to crush the rice grains.

Cool the rice by fanning it for a minute or two, then gently fold the rice over and repeat the fanning until the rice has cooled to room temperature. Divide into four equal portions.

Now make the rolls. A sushi mat makes things much easier, but if you don't have one, a piece of parchment paper can be used to help form the rolls. The rice will be very sticky so have a bowl of water ready to dip your fingers into.

Place one of the nori sheets shiny side down on the sushi mat with the long edge horizontal. With damp fingers, spread one portion of the rice evenly over the sheet, leaving a ¾-inch gap along the top edge. Place strips of smoked salmon in a horizontal line on top of the rice about ½-inch from the bottom edge, followed by a line

of cucumber strips, a line of carrot strips and a small amount of wasabi (if using).

Run a wet finger over the top edge of the nori and start rolling the mat away from you, using it to compress the filling inside gently. Make a join along the top dampened edge.

Place the roll on a chopping board and, using a very sharp knife, trim the edges and slice the roll into six pieces. Repeat with the other nori sheets. Pour the soy or teriyaki dipping sauce into a small bowl and serve with the sushi rolls.

Chosen as a source of: vitamins, B12, D, fish/seafood / Per 12 pieces: 290 kcal; 2.4g fat; 0.3g saturated fat / 0.5 portions of fruit/vegetables

soy seared tuna

Fresh tuna has a lovely firm texture and is a good fish to try if you haven't previously been keen on fish. Sesame oil adds a great depth of flavor.

SERVES 2

2 fresh tuna steaks (each about 4½ ounces)

For the marinade
¼ cup orange juice
¼ cup light soy sauce
1 teaspoon toasted sesame oil

1 tablespoon olive oil
1 teaspoon sesame seeds
1 garlic clove, finely chopped
Zest of ½ orange
1 tablespoon chopped fresh dill, or 1 teaspoon dried

Combine all the marinade ingredients in a bowl and mix well.

Place the tuna steaks into a shallow dish, coat well in the marinade, cover and marinate for 1–2 hours.

Heat a nonstick pan over medium heat and sear the tuna for 2 minutes on each side (or until cooked to your liking). Serve with a wedge of lemon, some boiled baby potatoes and a simple green side salad like the one on page 137.

You could use this marinade for any firm fish or even chicken.

Chosen as a source of: vitamins B6, B12, C, D, selenium, MUFA, fish/seafood / Per serving: 258 kcal; 14.9g fat; 2.7g saturated fat

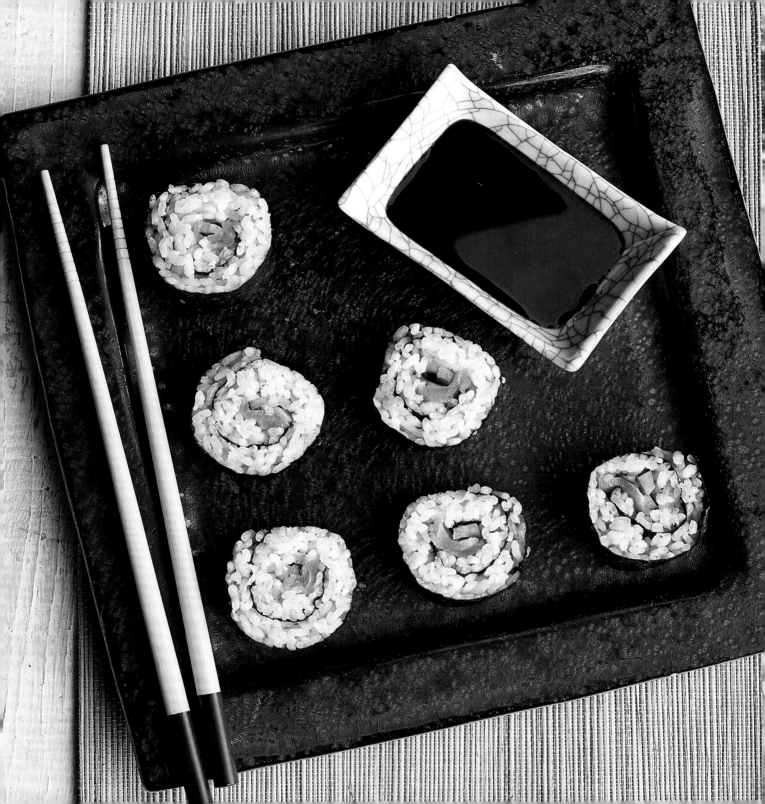

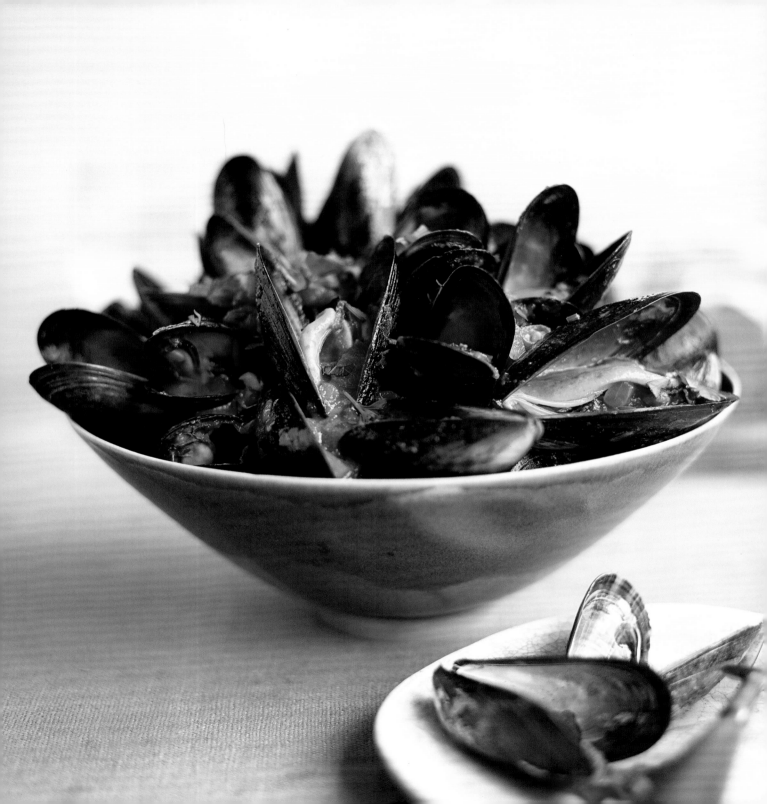

mussels marinara

This is a quick and easy recipe for mussels. The key to this dish is to use a good-quality white wine. Serve with fresh wholegrain crusty bread.

SERVES 2

1 pound 2 ounces mussels
1 tablespoon olive oil
1 onion, finely chopped
2 small garlic cloves, crushed or finely chopped
½ teaspoon dried oregano
½ fresh red chili, finely chopped or ¼ teaspoon dried chili flakes (optional)

½ cup good-quality dry white wine
14-ounce can chopped tomatoes
2 tablespoons roughly chopped flat-leaf parsley

Clean and debeard the mussels, discarding any with broken shells or any that do not close when tapped on the countertop.

Heat the olive oil in a large pan and cook the onion, garlic, oregano and chili, if using, over medium heat until the onion is soft and translucent.

Add the wine and bring to a boil. Add the tomatoes and half the parsley and simmer for 3–4 minutes.

Tip in the mussels and simmer for another 3–4 minutes until the shells open. Discard any unopened mussels. Serve the mussels with the remaining parsley sprinkled over the top.

Chosen as a source of: vitamins B6, B12, C, E, folate, selenium, fish/seafood, polyphenols / Per serving: 236 kcal; 8.6g fat; 1.2g saturated fat / 3 portions of fruit/vegetables

chermoula shrimp

Chermoula paste is used in North African cooking and usually includes garlic, cilantro, lemon, olive oil and spices. We have used it here as a sauce for shrimp, but it works just as well with other fish or meat. Serve these as part of a meze or team with rice and a salad to make a more substantial meal.

SERVES 4

½ tablespoon olive oil, for frying
14 ounces shrimp, peeled and deveined (leave the tails on for decoration)

For the chermoula
2 garlic cloves, crushed or finely chopped
Zest of ½ lemon
2 tablespoons lemon juice

3 tablespoons freshly chopped flat-leaf parsley
3 tablespoons freshly chopped cilantro
1 teaspoon paprika
½ teaspoon chili flakes or ½ fresh red chili (optional)
½ teaspoon cumin
3 tablespoons olive oil

To make the chermoula, place the garlic, lemon zest and juice, herbs and spices and 1 tablespoon of the olive oil in a small food-processor (or pestle and mortar) and process briefly. Continue to add the remaining olive oil slowly while processing until well combined.

Heat the ½ tablespoon of oil in a pan and fry the shrimp over medium heat until just turning pink, then add the chermoula, coating the shrimp well, and continue to cook for 2–3 minutes until the shrimp are firm.

Chermoula is very versatile. You can use it to marinate skewers of lamb or chicken breast for a couple of hours before barbecuing, or spread it on fish fillets before baking.

Chosen as a source of: vitamins B12, C, E, selenium, MUFA, fish/seafood, polyphenols / Per serving: 183 kcal; 11.8g fat; 1.7g saturated fat

linguine with garlic, shrimp and spinach

Many thanks to Gino D'Acampo for sharing this recipe, originally published in his book *The Italian Diet*. This is a delicious, quick and easy dish that requires minimal preparation.

SERVES 4

10½ ounces linguine
4 tablespoons extra virgin
  olive oil
2–3 garlic cloves, sliced
5½ ounces spinach leaves
14 ounces raw shrimp, peeled
4 tablespoons freshly chopped
  flat-leaf parsley

10 cherry tomatoes, halved or
  quartered
Zest of 1 lemon
Salt and freshly ground black
  pepper

Cook the pasta in a large pan of boiling, salted water according to the package instructions or until *al dente*.

While the pasta is cooking, heat the oil in a large frying pan over medium heat. Add the garlic and fry gently for 1 minute. Add the spinach and cook for 2 more minutes.

Add the shrimp along with the parsley and season with black pepper and salt if required. Stir well and continue to cook for 2–3 minutes.

Drain the pasta and add to the frying pan with the cherry tomatoes and lemon zest. Stir together for 30 seconds then serve immediately.

Although raw shrimp will give the best results, you could use cooked shrimp if you prefer.

Chosen as a source of: vitamins B6, B12, C, E, folate, selenium, MUFA, fish/seafood, polyphenols / Per serving: 467 kcal; 15.2g fat; 2.2g saturated fat / 1 portion of fruit/vegetables

seared scallops with walnut salsa verde

Thank you to chef and author Dale Pinnock, who kindly provided this recipe—full of fresh flavors and textures.

SERVES 2

Olive oil, for frying
5–6 large scallops (without roe)
Mixed salad leaves, to serve

For the salsa verde
1 tablespoon white wine vinegar
A small bunch of fresh flat-leaf
  parsley
A small bunch of fresh mint
1 tablespoon capers
1 tablespoon chopped walnuts
5 anchovy fillets
1½ tablespoons olive oil

Place all the ingredients for the salsa in a food-processor. Process on very low speed in order to retain a coarse, "chunky" consistency. You may wish to add a little more oil, depending on how thick or loose you like it.

Heat a little olive oil in a frying pan over medium heat. Add the scallops and fry for about 3 minutes on each side.

Lay the scallops over some mixed salad greens, and serve with the salsa verde.

Chosen as a source of: vitamins, B12, C, E, folate, selenium, MUFA, fish/seafood, polyphenols / Per serving: 335 kcal; 22g fat; 2.7g saturated fat / 0.5 portions of fruit/vegetables

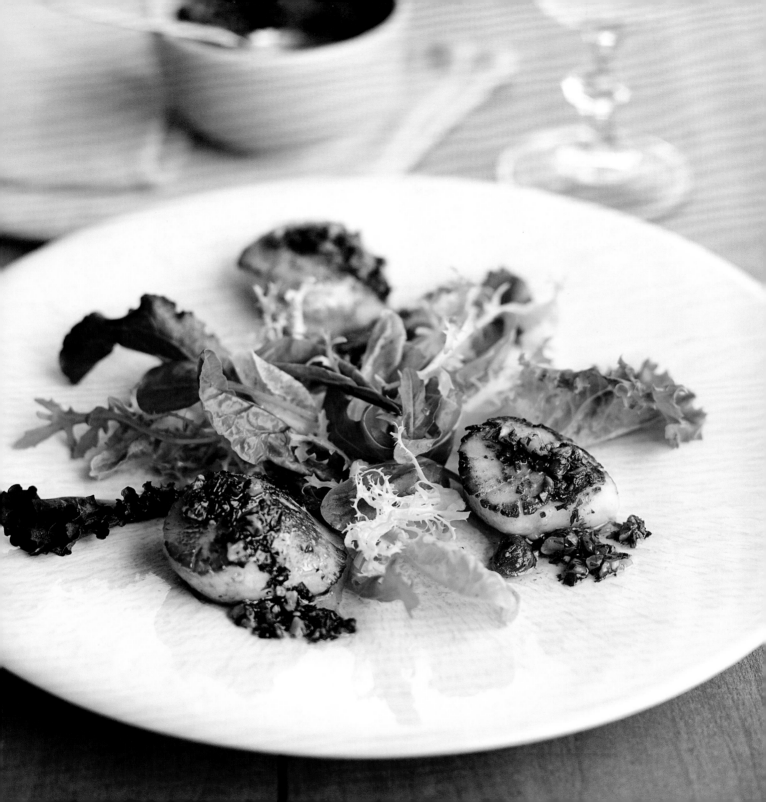

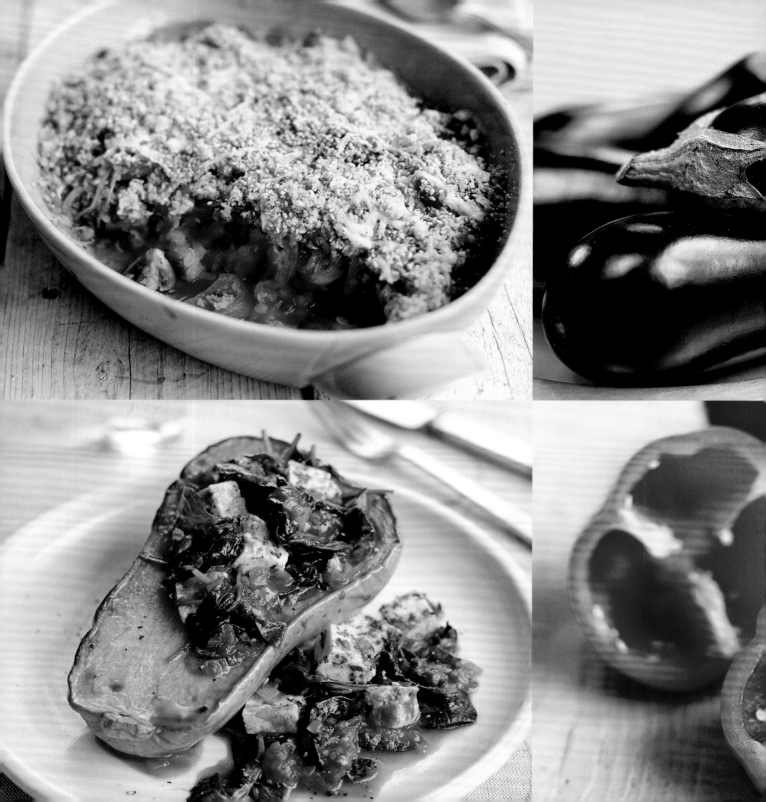

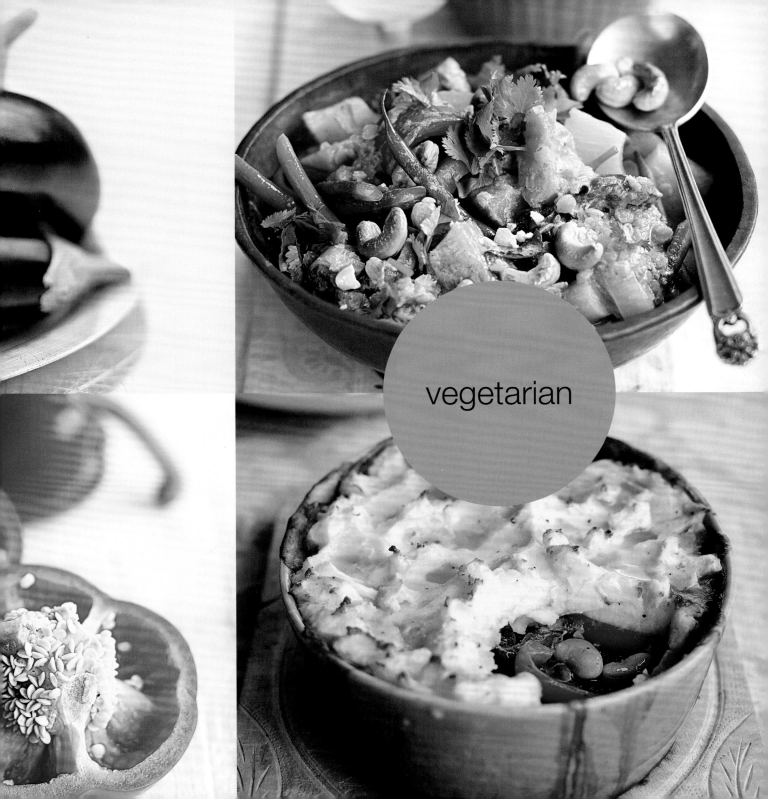

vegetarian

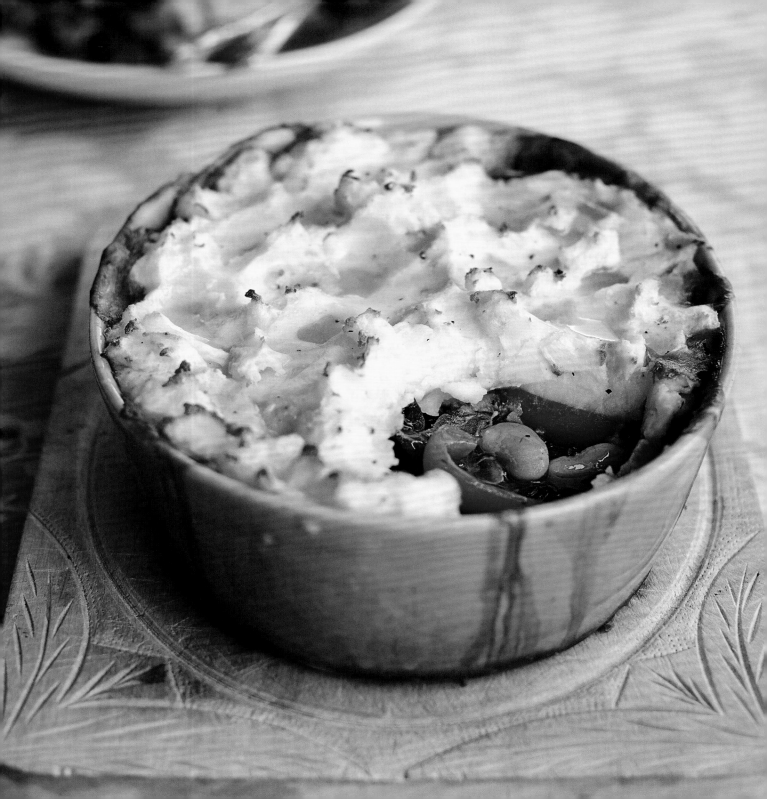

leek and lima bean pie

Packed with colorful vegetables in a luscious cider sauce, this delicious pie is the ultimate in comfort food for a cold day.

SERVES 4

1 tablespoon canola oil, plus extra for greasing
2–3 leeks (about 12 ounces), washed and sliced
1 large red pepper, seeded and sliced
7 ounces mushrooms, washed and halved
14-ounce can lima beans, drained
Generous 1 cup vegetable stock made with 1 stock cube
Scant 1 cup medium dry hard cider
1–2 teaspoons dried sage
3 tablespoons cornstarch
1 pound 10 ounces mashed potato or cooled, boiled potatoes that have been thickly sliced
A drizzle of garlic-infused olive oil
Freshly ground black pepper

Preheat the oven to 350°F and grease a large baking dish with a little oil.

Heat the tablespoon of canola oil in a large pan over medium heat. Add the leeks, red pepper and mushrooms and cook gently for about 5 minutes until beginning to soften.

Add the lima beans, stock, cider and sage and bring to a boil. Reduce the heat and simmer gently, covered, for about 15 minutes. Mix the cornstarch with a little cold water to make a paste and then add a ladleful of the hot liquid and stir well. Transfer the loosened paste to the pan and stir through to thicken the sauce. Season with black pepper and then transfer to the prepared baking dish.

Spread the mashed potato or arrange overlapping potato slices evenly on top of the pie filling. Drizzle with a little garlic-infused olive oil and bake in the oven, uncovered, for about 20–25 minutes until the potatoes are golden and turning crunchy and the filling is starting to bubble through the topping.

Serve with seasonal green vegetables such as broccoli, asparagus, kale or zucchini.

Chosen as a source of: vitamins B6, C, E, folate, pulses, polyphenols / Per serving: 306 kcal; 6.7g fat; 1g saturated fat / 3 portions of fruit/vegetables

red wine casserole

This is a lovely light, fragrant dish and a really good way to include some beans in a meal. It takes hardly any time to cook compared to a meat-based casserole, yet is still full of flavor and extremely satisfying.

SERVES 4

1 tablespoon canola oil
2 carrots, sliced
1 large red pepper, seeded and thickly sliced
1 large red onion, chopped
14-ounce can red kidney beans, drained
9 ounces cauliflower florets
5½ ounces chestnut mushrooms, halved or thickly sliced
9 ounces canned apricots in juice
Generous 1 cup red wine
Generous 1 cup vegetable stock made with 1 stock cube
Zest of 1 lemon
1 tablespoon arrowroot or cornstarch
Salt and freshly ground black pepper

Heat the canola oil in a large pan over medium heat. Add the carrots, peppers and onion and cook gently for 5 minutes until starting to soften.

Add the rest of the ingredients except the cornstarch or arrowroot to the pan. Bring to a boil, lower the heat and simmer, covered, for 20 minutes.

Season to taste. Mix the arrowroot or cornstarch with a little cold water to make a paste and then add a ladleful of the hot liquid and stir well. Transfer the loosened paste to the pan and stir through to thicken the sauce.

Serve immediately with rice and green vegetables or salad.

Kidney beans go especially well with the red wine sauce but you could also try using cannellini or pinto beans for a change.

Chosen as a source of: vitamins B6, C, folate, pulses, polyphenols / Per serving: 262 kcal; 4.9g fat; 0.5g saturated fat / 4.5 portions of fruit/vegetables

roasted mediterranean butternut squash

This is a really good recipe to introduce people who think they don't like it to tofu. The Italian herb variety is now available in most supermarkets and complements the savory tomato and sweet butternut in this substantial and colorful dish.

SERVES 4

2 small butternut squash (about 2¼ pounds total weight), washed, halved lengthwise, and seeded
1 tablespoon garlic-infused olive oil

1 quantity of Tasty Tomato Sauce (page 145)
2 teaspoons dried oregano
14 ounces Italian herb tofu, cubed
12 ounces spinach leaves
Freshly ground black pepper

Preheat the oven to 400°F.

Brush the butternut halves inside and out with garlic-infused oil and season with black pepper. Place cut-side down on a baking sheet and roast for 20 minutes or until the squash is tender all the way through.

Heat the tomato sauce in a large pan and stir in the oregano. Add the tofu and simmer gently for 5 minutes. Add the spinach, cover, and leave to simmer for 2–3 minutes. Remove the lid and stir through the wilted spinach leaves.

Place one butternut half per person on a plate and spoon the tomato and tofu sauce on top. Serve with green vegetables or salad and crusty bread.

The tomato and tofu sauce is delicious stirred through cooked pasta. It also makes a great topping for a baked potato.

Per serving: 241 kcal; 9.9g fat; 1.3g saturated fat / Chosen as a source of: vitamins B6, C, E, folate, soy, polyphenols / 4 portions of fruit/vegetables

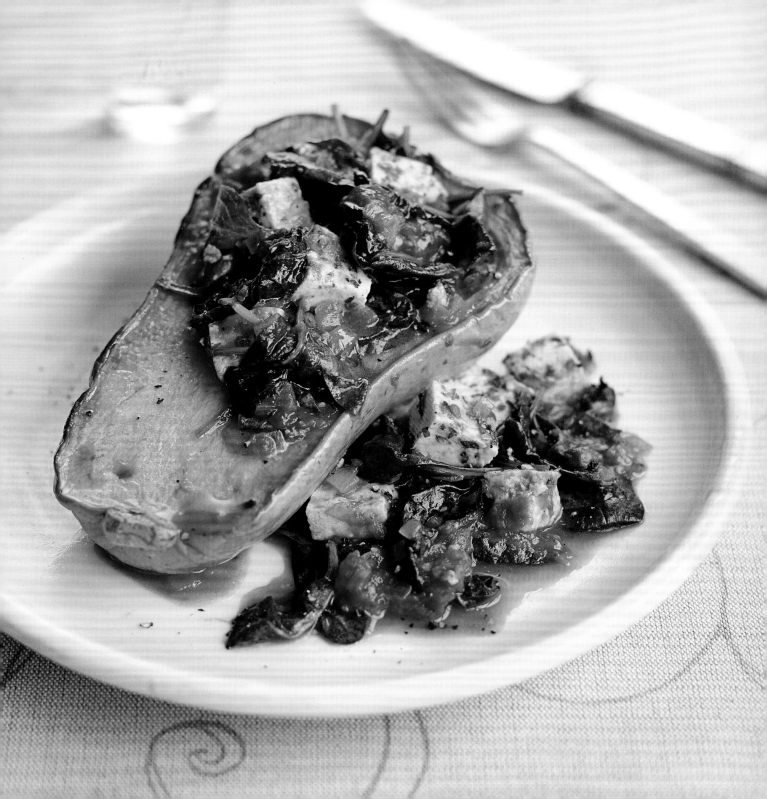

roasted vegetable frittata

It's amazing how a few simple ingredients can combine to make something really special. If you are not keen on cheese, it can be omitted.

SERVES 4–6

1 red onion, cut into wedges
1 small eggplant, cubed
2 zucchini, chopped
1 orange pepper, seeded and cut into chunks
A handful of fresh woody herbs such as rosemary or thyme, or 1–2 teaspoons dried Mediterranean herbs
1 tablespoon garlic-infused olive oil
2 raw beets, trimmed and peeled
5½ ounces chestnut mushrooms, halved
5½ ounces cherry tomatoes, halved

1 tablespoon canola oil
8 large free-range eggs, lightly beaten
Scant 1 cup skim milk
A small handful of fresh herbs, such as parsley or chives
4½ ounces low-fat mozzarella, torn into chunks, or 2¾ ounces low-fat Cheddar, grated, or 1 ounce (about ⅓ cup) coarsely grated Parmesan
Torn basil leaves, to garnish
Salt and freshly ground black pepper

Preheat the oven to 400°F and line a large baking sheet with parchment paper.

Toss the onion, eggplant, zucchini, pepper and herbs in a bowl with the garlic oil and arrange on the baking sheet. Toss the beets in the remaining oil and add to the baking sheet. Tossing it separately stops it from "staining" the rest of the vegetables. Roast for 15 minutes, then add the mushrooms and tomatoes and return to the oven for a further 10 minutes.

Heat the canola oil in a large (11-inch) nonstick frying pan and add the roasted vegetables to the pan. Mix the beaten eggs with the milk and herbs and season. Pour into the pan on top of the vegetables. Cook over low–medium heat for about 10 minutes; meanwhile, preheat the broiler to high.

Arrange your chosen cheese on top of the frittata. Cook under the preheated broiler until the top is golden brown and gently set. Cut the frittata into wedges and serve garnished with a few torn basil leaves. Delicious served hot or cold.

Chosen as a source of: vitamins B6, B12, C, D, E, folate, selenium, MUFA, polyphenols / Per serving (based on 4 servings): 337 kcal; 22g fat; 5.9g saturated fat / 3.5 portions of fruit/vegetables

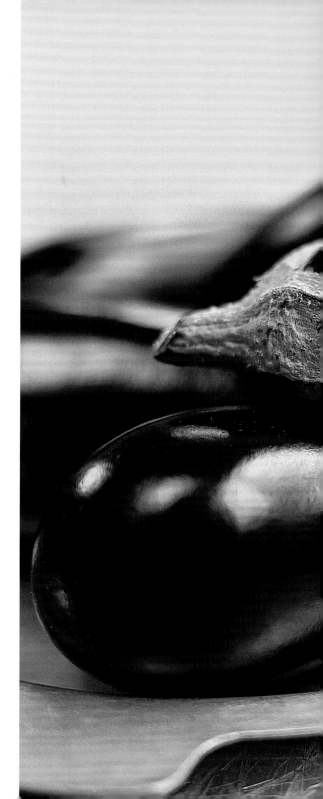

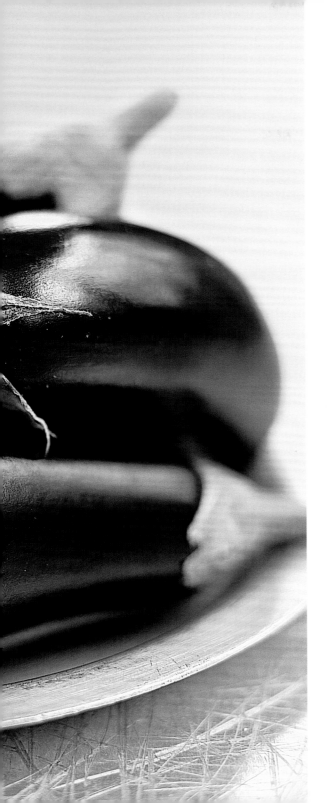

eggplant pasticcio

A traditional dish that has been a firm favorite for years. It freezes well and can be reheated with no loss of flavor.

SERVES 4–6

8 ounces quick-cook macaroni
1 red onion, chopped
1 red pepper, seeded and chopped
1 large eggplant, trimmed and cubed
2 garlic cloves, crushed
2 tablespoons olive oil

½ quantity of Tasty Tomato Sauce (page 145)
¼ cup pitted black olives, sliced
¼ cup pitted green olives, sliced
2 free-range eggs, beaten
1 cup nonfat Greek yogurt
2¾ ounces low-fat feta cheese, crumbled
Freshly ground black pepper

Preheat the broiler to high and the oven to 375°F.

Cook the macaroni according to the package instructions or until *al dente*. Drain and set aside.

Toss the onion, pepper, eggplant and garlic in the olive oil and spread out on a baking sheet. Broil for about 10 minutes, turning occasionally, until charred.

Mix together the cooked macaroni, charred vegetables, tomato sauce and sliced olives and transfer to a large baking dish.

Stir together the eggs, yogurt and feta and season with some black pepper. Pour the mixture over the macaroni, then bake in the oven for 20–25 minutes until the topping is lightly set and golden. Serve with a green salad.

If you don't have time to make the tomato sauce, using a jar of shop-bought tomato and olive pasta sauce also produces good results.

Chosen as a source of: vitamins B6, B12, C, E, folate, selenium, MUFA, polyphenols / Per serving (based on 4 servings): 464 kcal; 17.4g fat; 3.7g saturated fat / 3 portions of fruit/vegetables

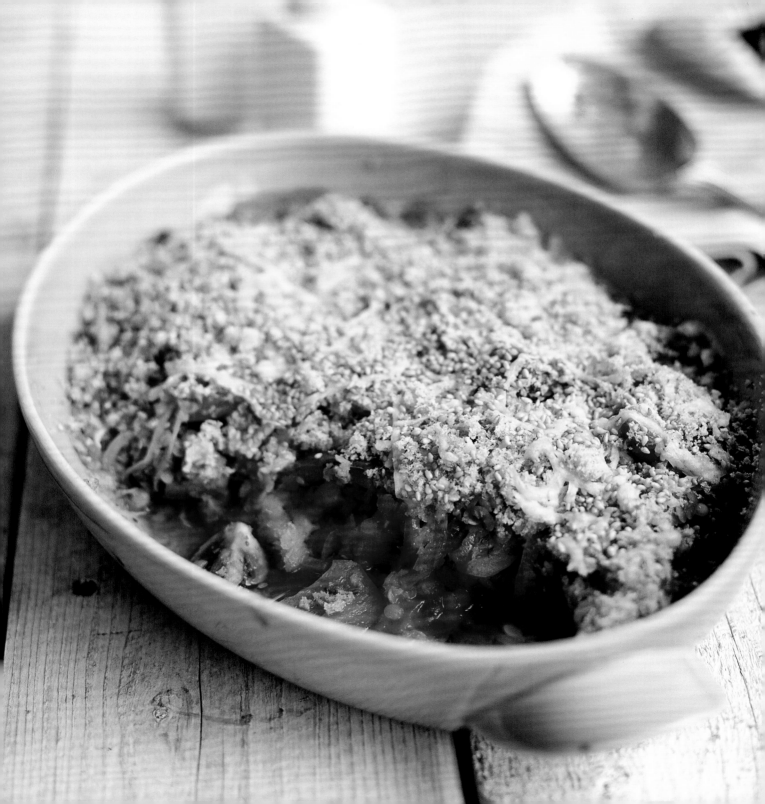

lentil and mushroom bake

Thank you to Wayne Robinson, Head Chef at the Royal Berkshire Hospital in Reading, for sharing this recipe with us. This popular and tasty dish has been a firm favorite with both staff and patients in the hospital restaurant and on the wards.

SERVES 4

5¾ ounces (1 cup) red lentils
1 tablespoon canola oil
2 onions, finely sliced
1 red and 1 green pepper, seeded and chopped
2 garlic cloves, peeled and crushed
3½ ounces chestnut mushrooms
3 tablespoons tomato paste
1¼ cups vegetable stock made with 1 stock cube

1–2 teaspoons dried mixed herbs
2¾ ounces low-fat Cheddar cheese, grated
1¾ ounces (about 1 cup) wholewheat breadcrumbs
2 tablespoons sesame seeds
Salt and freshly ground black pepper

Preheat the oven to 300°F and lightly grease a baking dish.

Put the lentils in a pan and cover with cold water. Bring to a boil, simmer for 5 minutes, then drain and set aside.

Heat the canola oil in a large pan over medium heat. Add the onions, peppers and garlic and cook gently for 5 minutes until beginning to soften.

Add the mushrooms, tomato paste, stock and mixed herbs with a good grinding of black pepper and a little salt if required. Bring to a boil, stir, add the lentils, and simmer for 5–10 minutes.

Transfer the mixture to the prepared dish. Mix together the cheese, breadcrumbs and sesame seeds and scatter over the top. Bake in the oven for about 30 minutes until the topping is golden. Serve with salad or green vegetables.

Try substituting white wine or hard cider for the stock to give a fruitier taste.

Chosen as a source of: vitamins B6, C, E, folate, pulses, polyphenols / Per serving: 374 kcal; 11.4g fat; 3g saturated fat / 3 portions of fruit/ vegetables

mushroom and tomato risotto

This is a lower-fat version of traditional risotto, but still has a deep, rich flavor thanks to the dried mushrooms and Parmesan.

SERVES 2

½ ounce sun-dried shiitake mushrooms
¾ ounce sun-dried tomatoes
1 tablespoon olive oil
1 onion, finely chopped
1 large garlic clove, finely chopped
3½ ounces fresh chestnut mushrooms, sliced

Generous ¾ cup risotto rice (e.g. Arborio or carnaroli)
½ cup good-quality dry white wine
2 cups vegetable stock
1 ounce Parmesan cheese, grated
A large handful of freshly chopped flat-leaf parsley

Soak the dried shiitake mushrooms and sun-dried tomatoes in boiling water for about 10–20 minutes until soft and then drain.

Heat the oil in a pan and gently cook the onion and garlic until translucent. Add the fresh chestnut mushrooms and cook for 2–3 minutes.

Add the rice, stirring to coat the grains in the oil, and sauté for 2–3 minutes. Add the wine and cook for another 3 minutes, then add the tomatoes and shiitake mushrooms. Add a ladleful of stock at a time, stirring continuously until the stock is absorbed, before adding the next ladleful. Continue until all the stock is used up and the rice is cooked but still retains some bite. Add a little warm water if more liquid is needed.

Stir in half of the Parmesan and all the parsley, then sprinkle with the remaining Parmesan and serve.

Chosen as a source of: vitamins B6, D, C, folate, selenium, polyphenols / Per serving: 521 kcal; 11.9g fat; 4.1g saturated fat / 2 portions of fruit/ vegetables

soybean patties

Vibrant green, with a slightly soft consistency, these make a good alternative to a meat burger patty served in a bun. Alternatively, simply serve with a Mango or Tomato and Pepper Salsa (page 143).

SERVES 2 AS A MAIN OR 4 AS AN APPETIZER

1 small–medium potato, peeled and quartered
5½ ounces frozen soybeans
½ x 14-ounce can cannellini beans, drained
2 scallions, finely chopped
1 teaspoon paprika

A good handful of finely chopped cilantro
6 tablespoons (1½ ounces) cornmeal, for coating
2 tablespoons canola oil
Salt and freshly ground black pepper

Boil the potato in water for 15 minutes or until soft enough to mash. Mash well and then place in a large bowl.

Cook the soybeans in boiling water for 1–2 minutes until just soft. Add to the bowl along with the cannellini beans, scallions, paprika, cilantro and salt and pepper and mash together. You are aiming for the result to be smooth enough to form a patty, but still have some bits for texture.

Form the mixture into four patties and roll in the cornmeal to coat. Chill in the refrigerator for at least 30 minutes.

Heat the oil in a frying pan and fry the patties for 2–3 minutes each side until golden.

Chosen as a source of: vitamins B6, C, E, folate, MUFA, soy, pulses, polyphenols / Per serving (based on 2 servings): 596 kcal; 28g fat; 3.1g saturated fat / 2 portions of fruit/vegetables

thai green vegetable curry

The addition of sweet pineapple to this vibrant curry gives it a real lift. The green chili adds a little extra heat but this can be left out if you prefer a more subtly spiced dish.

SERVES 6

1 tablespoon canola oil
2 echalion (banana) shallots, chopped
1 green chili, seeded and finely chopped
2 ounces Thai green curry paste
2¾ ounces (½ cup) red lentils
2 leeks, washed and sliced
1 red and 1 yellow pepper, seeded and thickly sliced
10½ ounces butternut squash, peeled and cubed
7 ounces green beans, trimmed and cut into 1¼-inch lengths

1¼ cups low-fat coconut milk
8-ounce can pineapple slices, drained and cut into chunks
5½ ounces spinach leaves
Salt and freshly ground black pepper

To garnish
A large handful of fresh cilantro, chopped
2¾ ounces (about ⅔ cup) cashews, toasted in a dry pan

Heat the canola oil in a large, nonstick pan over low–medium heat. Add the shallots and green chili and cook gently for a few minutes. Add the green curry paste and cook gently for a further 2 minutes, stirring frequently.

Stir the lentils into the paste then add the leeks, peppers, squash, beans and coconut milk. Bring to a boil then lower the heat and simmer, covered, for about 20 minutes, by which time the lentils should be very soft.

Stir in the pineapple pieces and add the spinach leaves. Cover the pan and simmer for 2 more minutes, by which time the spinach will have wilted and can be stirred easily into the sauce.

Taste and adjust the seasoning. Serve with Thai jasmine rice and top with the fresh cilantro and toasted cashews.

Sweet potato or even pumpkin can be used in place of butternut squash.

Chosen as a source of: vitamins B6, C, E, folate, pulses, polyphenols / Per serving: 262 kcal; 13.2g fat; 4.7g saturated fat / 3.5 portions of fruit/vegetables

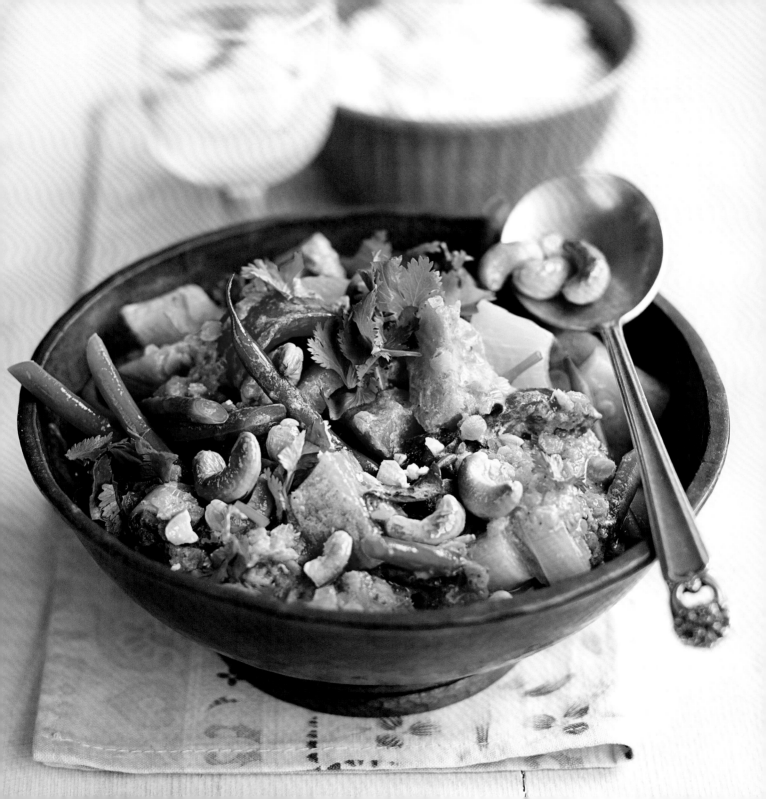

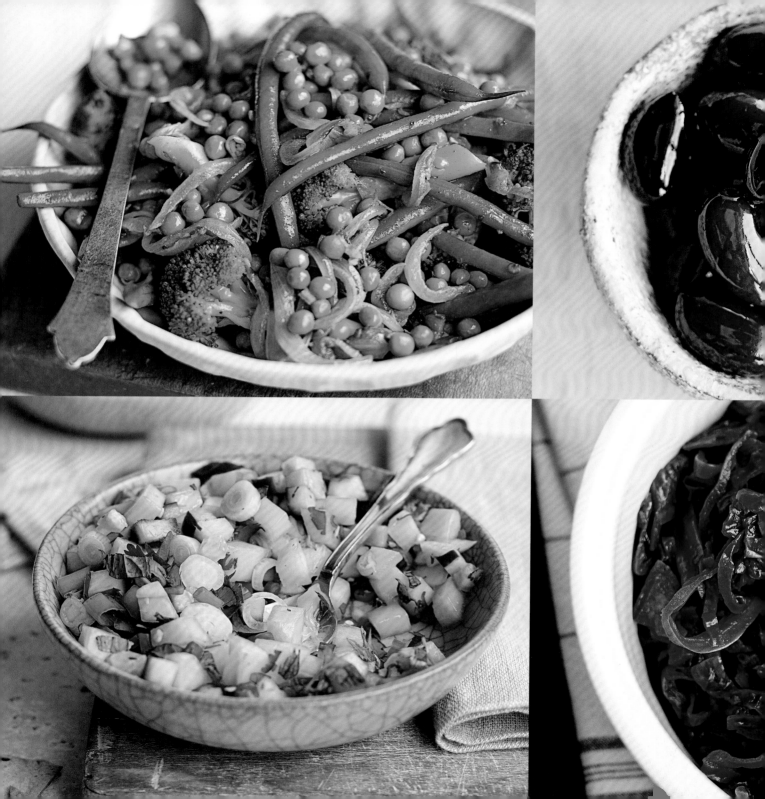

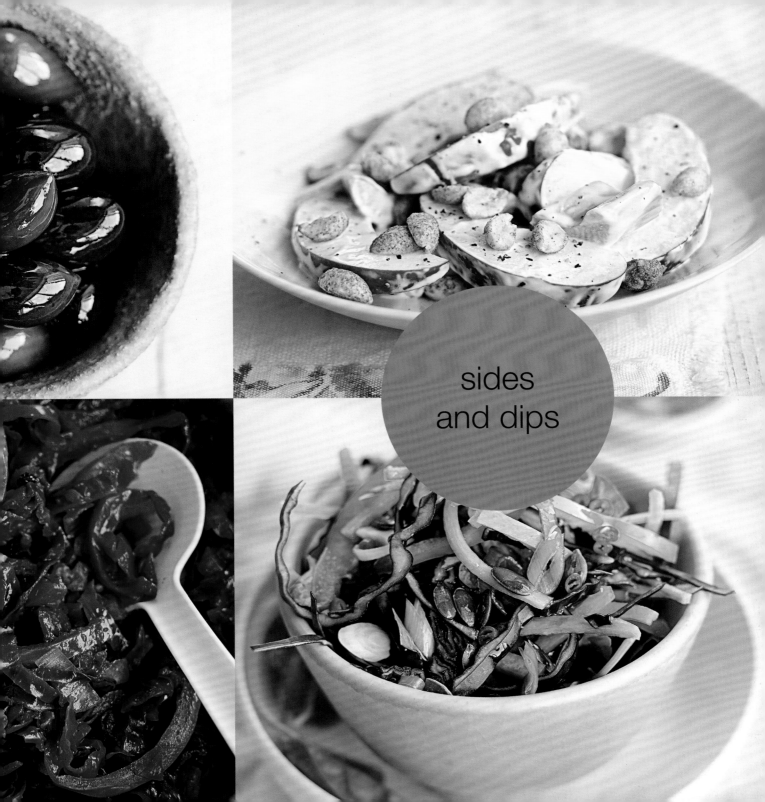

sides
and dips

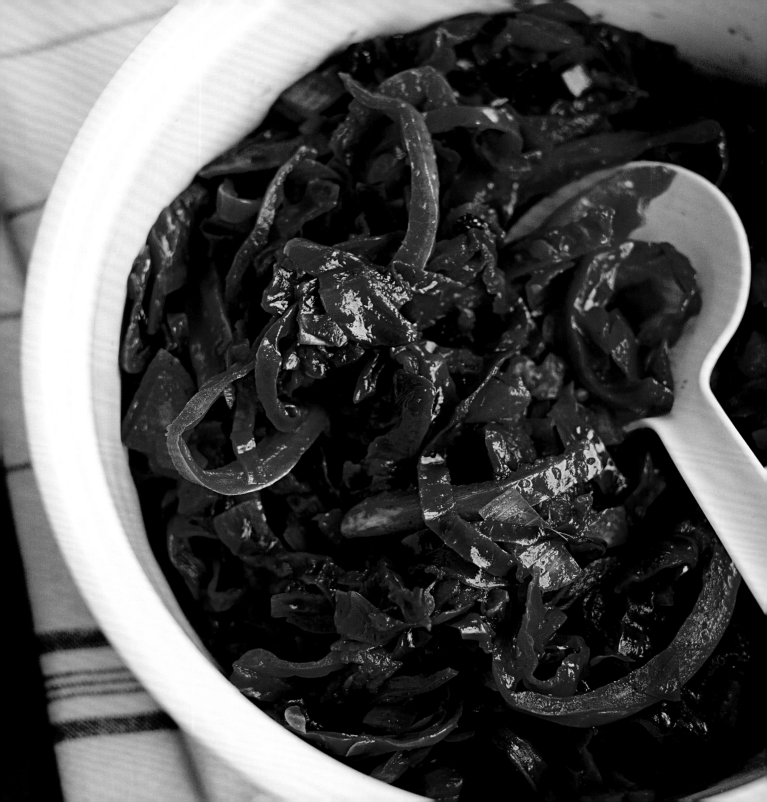

braised red cabbage with cider

This is a variation on a traditional spiced cabbage recipe. It makes a great accompaniment to roast pork, braised liver or cold turkey. The cabbage can be frozen in individual portions and reheated in the microwave without any harm.

SERVES 6

1 pound 10 ounces red cabbage, trimmed and thinly sliced
1 large onion, thinly sliced
2 medium cooking apples, peeled, cored and thinly sliced
About ½ cup raisins
1¾ cups medium/dry hard cider
Salt and freshly ground black pepper

Preheat the oven to 350°F.

Layer the cabbage, onion, apples and raisins in a flameproof casserole dish. Pour the cider over and add plenty of ground black pepper and a little salt.

Place the casserole over medium heat and heat gently until the cider is boiling. Transfer to the oven, tightly covered, and cook for about 1 hour, removing the casserole halfway through cooking to mix the ingredients together.

When the cabbage is tender, remove from the oven and stir again. Taste and adjust the seasoning, and serve.

Chosen as a source of: vitamins B6, C, folate, polyphenols / Per serving: 109 kcal; 0.5g fat; 0g saturated fat / 3 portions of fruit/vegetables

red cabbage and apple salad

Crunchy and fresh-flavored, this salad is delicious with cold meats or fish or as a side dish at a barbecue.

SERVES 4–6

4 red-skinned dessert apples
½ red cabbage, trimmed and finely shredded
1 large carrot, cut into matchsticks
⅓ cup raisins
A large handful of fresh flat-leaf parsley, roughly chopped

For the dressing
2½ tablespoons olive oil
1 tablespoon walnut oil
1½ tablespoons red wine vinegar
1½ tablespoons balsamic vinegar
Salt and freshly ground black pepper

Core, but do not peel, the apples. Cut each one into about 10–12 wedges and add to a large serving dish with the shredded cabbage, carrot and raisins.

Combine all the dressing ingredients in a screw-top jar and shake well to combine. Pour over the salad, toss gently to combine and leave to marinate for up to 30 minutes.

Stir in the chopped parsley just before serving.

Chosen as a source of: vitamin C, MUFA, polyphenols / Per serving (based on 4 servings): 245 kcal; 15.4g fat; 1.9g saturated fat / 2.5 portions of fruit/vegetables

spinach and pine nuts

Spinach is so quick to cook and when teamed with garlic and pine nuts makes an easy side to serve with fish or meat dishes.

SERVES 4

7 ounces spinach, washed and stalks removed
2 tablespoons olive oil
3 garlic cloves, finely sliced
1 ounce (about 3 tablespoons) pine nuts
Salt and freshly ground black pepper

Dry the spinach, either in a salad spinner or with paper towels.

Heat the oil in a large, lidded pan over low–medium heat. Add the garlic and pine nuts and cook over gentle heat, being careful not to let them burn. Add the spinach and toss gently to coat in the oil. Cover and let cook over low–medium heat for 1 minute. Toss again, cover and cook for a further minute. You want the spinach to be just wilted.

Season to taste and serve immediately.

Combine this with the Tasty Tomato Sauce on page 145 for a great sauce to stir through cooked pasta.

Chosen as a source of: vitamins C, E, folate, polyphenols / Per serving: 122 kcal; 11.7g fat; 1.3g saturated fat / 0.5 portion of fruit/vegetables

spiced green vegetables

This delicious alternative to plain boiled vegetables makes a great accompaniment to most of the fish dishes in this book.

SERVES 4

1½ tablespoons olive oil
1 onion, very finely sliced
1–2 garlic cloves, finely sliced
½ fresh red chili, seeded if preferred, or ¼ teaspoon dried chili flakes
1 teaspoon ground cumin
5¾ ounces fine green beans, topped and tailed and sliced on the diagonal
5¾ ounces (about 1¼ cups) frozen peas, defrosted
11¼ ounces broccoli, broken into small florets

Heat the oil in a large frying pan over medium heat. Add the onion and cook until translucent, about 5 minutes.

Add the garlic, chili and cumin and continue to cook until the onions are crispy.

Add the beans, peas and broccoli and stir-fry for 2–3 minutes or until the vegetables are just soft. Serve immediately.

You could use soybeans instead of the peas (blanch them before adding to the pan).

Chosen as a source of: vitamins B6, C, folate, pulses, polyphenols / Per serving: 123 kcal; 6.2g fat; 1g saturated fat / 2.5 portions of fruit/vegetables

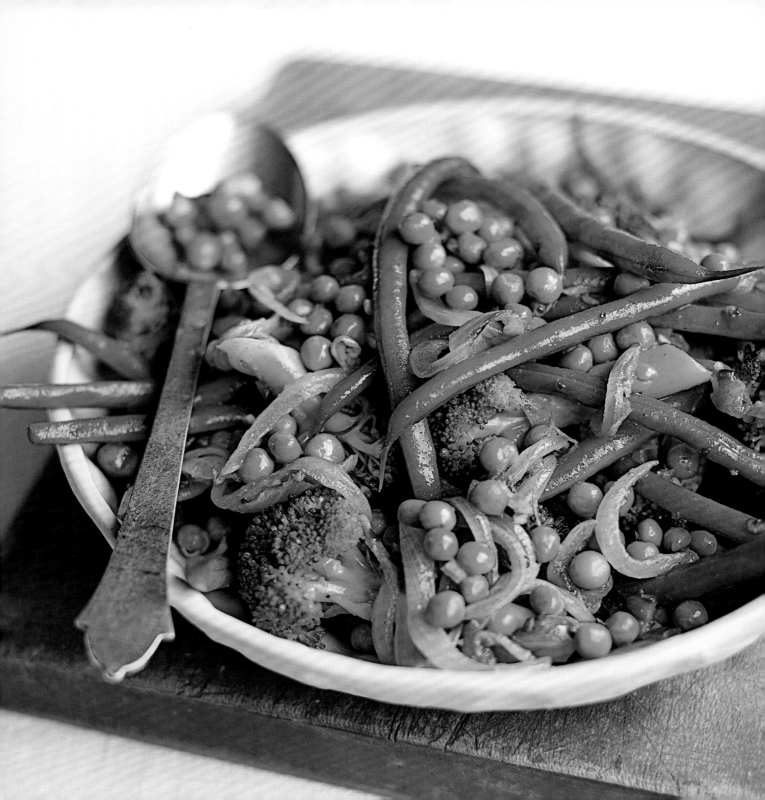

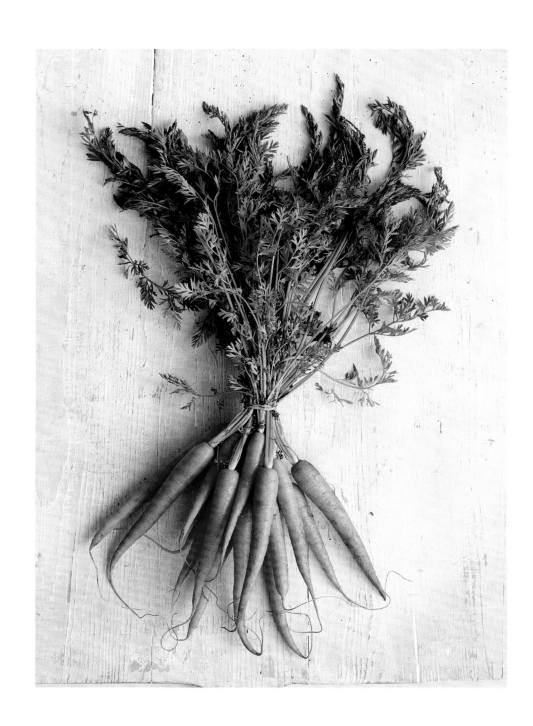

savory carrot salad

This carrot salad is simple to make and tastes even better the next day, once the flavors have had time to develop.

SERVES 4

2–3 large carrots, grated
1 medium beet, grated
A good handful of fresh
 cilantro, roughly chopped
A handful of walnuts, roughly
 chopped (optional)

For the dressing
1 tablespoon lemon juice
2 tablespoons orange juice
½ teaspoon ground cumin
½ tablespoon honey

Combine the dressing ingredients in a screw-top jar and shake well to combine; set aside.

Combine the carrots, beet, cilantro and walnuts (if using) in a salad bowl. Pour the dressing over the salad and stir well.

Chosen as a source of: vitamin C, folate, polyphenols / Per serving: 87 kcal; 5.4g fat; 0.5g saturated fat / 1 portion of fruit/vegetables

sweet carrot salad

A sweet version of the carrot salad, perfect as an accompaniment to lean cold meats or at a picnic or barbecue.

SERVES 4

2–3 large carrots, grated
1 medium beet, grated
A handful of walnuts, roughly
 chopped (optional)

8-ounce can pineapple slices
 in juice
1 tablespoon lemon juice

Place the carrots, beet and walnuts (if using) in a salad bowl.

Drain the pineapple, reserving the juice. Cut the pineapple into bite-size pieces and add these to the salad. Pour over the reserved juice and the lemon juice. Stir well.

Orange juice can be used instead of the drained pineapple juice if you find the salad too sweet. Canned mandarin pieces also work well.

Chosen as a source of: vitamin C, folate, polyphenols / Per serving: 129 kcal; 7.9g fat; 0.7g saturated fat / 1.5 portions of fruit/vegetables

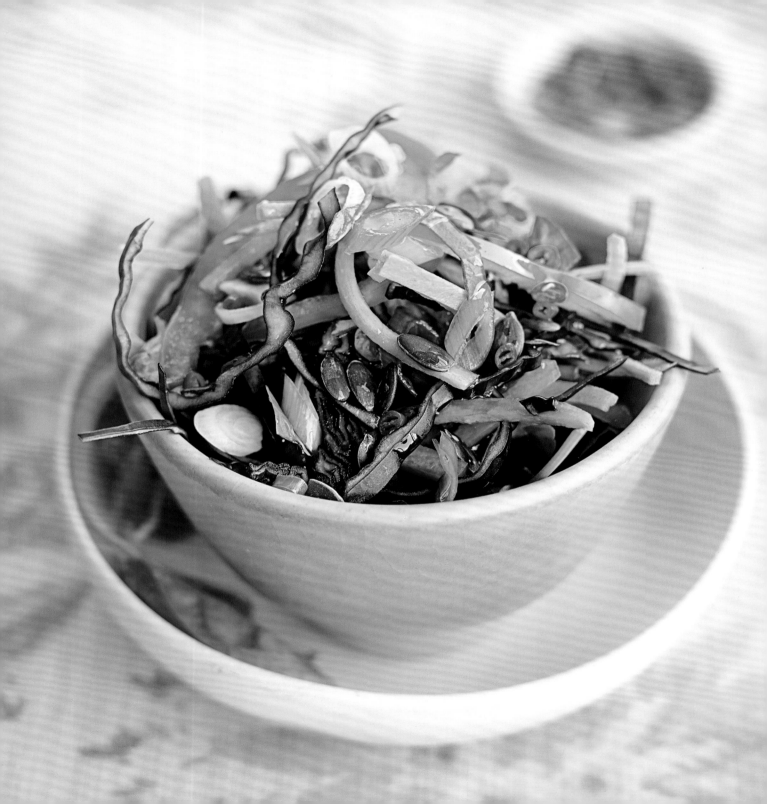

crunchy tricolor salad

Full of crisp, shredded vegetables, this is a healthy alternative to traditional coleslaw. It can be made a day ahead and stored in the refrigerator.

SERVES 6

2 carrots, cut into fine batons
7 ounces mixed spinach and arugula leaves, finely chopped
2 scallions, finely sliced on the diagonal
½ red cabbage, finely sliced
1 green pepper, seeded and finely sliced
A handful of pumpkin seeds

For the dressing
5 tablespoons olive oil
2 tablespoons red wine vinegar
1 tablespoon honey
½ red chili, seeded if preferred, and finely chopped, or ½ teaspoon chili flakes (optional)

Place all the dressing ingredients in a small pitcher or bowl and stir well to combine; set aside.

Combine all the salad ingredients, except the pumpkin seeds, in a large salad bowl. Pour the dressing over and toss to coat.

Sprinkle the pumpkin seeds over the top just before serving.

Chosen as a source of: vitamins, C, folate, MUFA, polyphenols / Per serving: 164 kcal; 12.9g fat; 1.7g saturated fat / 2 portions of fruit/vegetables

green leaf and herb salad

This is a very fresh-tasting green side salad full of different textures. Finish by sprinkling with a few pomegranate seed gems.

SERVES 4

3½ ounces mixed salad greens
A large handful of cilantro, roughly chopped
2 scallions, sliced on the diagonal
3-inch piece of cucumber, sliced and quartered
1 ripe avocado, peeled, pitted and cubed
½–¾ ounce (1½–2 tablespoons) pistachios, roughly chopped

1 tablespoon pomegranate seeds (optional)

For the dressing
3 tablespoons olive oil
1 tablespoon red wine vinegar
1 teaspoon honey
1½ tablespoons orange juice
½ teaspoon Dijon mustard

Combine all the salad ingredients except the pomegranate seeds in a large bowl.

Combine the dressing ingredients in a small pitcher or bowl and stir well to combine. Drizzle the dressing over the salad.

Sprinkle the pomegranate seeds over the top.

Chosen as a source of: vitamins C, E, polyphenols / Per serving: 129 kcal; 11.8g fat; 2.2g saturated fat / 1.5 portions of fruit/vegetables

mackerel pâté

You can make this pâté a day ahead; keep it refrigerated and serve with some dark rye bread and a side salad as a quick, light supper. It is also an easy way to incorporate some oily fish into your diet.

SERVES 4

5½ ounces smoked mackerel, skin removed	Juice of 1 lemon
3½ ounces (about ½ cup) very low-fat cream cheese	1 tablespoon finely chopped fresh dill (optional)
	Freshly ground black pepper

Break the fish up into small pieces to check for, and remove, any bones.

Place the fish, cream cheese, lemon juice, dill and some black pepper in a food-processor and blend until smooth. Taste and add more lemon juice and/or pepper if needed.

If you do not have a food-processor or prefer a more textured pâté, place all the ingredients in a bowl and mash well with a fork to the desired consistency.

For a stronger-flavored pâté, try using peppered mackerel fillets. Alternatively, replace the mackerel with smoked salmon and add a little parsley.

Chosen as a source of vitamins B12, D, fish/seafood / Per serving: 162 kcal; 12.8g fat; 3.2g saturated fat

celery, apple and peanut salad

This simple, tasty side dish is ready in a couple of minutes and is great served at a barbecue or with tomato-based dishes such as the Eggplant and Tomato Gratin on page 56.

SERVES 2

1 red-skinned dessert apple	1 tablespoon light mayonnaise
2–3 sticks celery, washed and cut into chunks	1 tablespoon nonfat Greek yogurt
1¾ ounces (about 1/3 cup) dry-roasted peanuts	Freshly ground black pepper

Cut the apple into quarters and remove the core but do not peel. Cut the quarters in half again and then cut into slim chunks. Place in a large bowl with the celery and peanuts.

Mix the mayonnaise and yogurt together with a good grinding of black pepper. Add to the bowl and mix through with a large spoon until everything is coated with the mayonnaise mixture. Serve immediately.

Substitute some toasted cashews for the peanuts.

Chosen as a source of: vitamin E, pulses, polyphenols / Per serving: 239 kcal; 17.3g fat; 2.9g saturated fat / 1.5 portions of fruit/vegetables

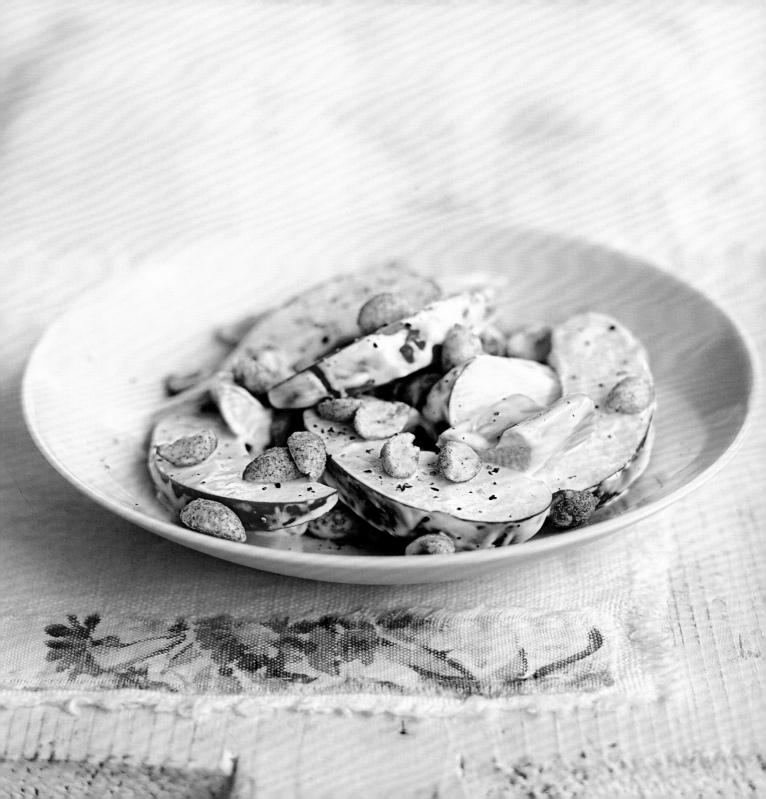

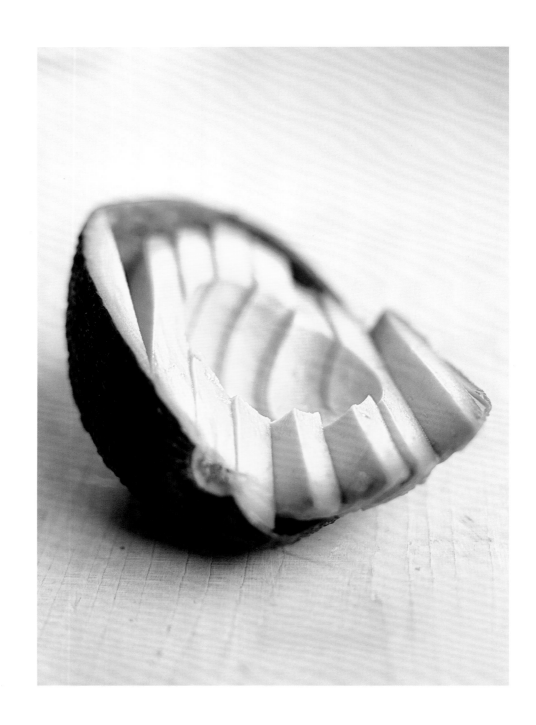

guacamole

This fresh guacamole can be used to add flavor to wraps or sandwiches or can be served as a dip for crudités of carrot, celery, cucumber or peppers. The lime should help to stop the avocado going brown, but it is best to eat this dip as soon as possible after making.

SERVES 4–6

2 ripe tomatoes, roughly chopped
1 small red onion, roughly chopped
1 small chili, seeded if preferred, finely chopped (add more or less to taste)
Juice of ½ lime

A handful of cilantro, roughly chopped
2 ripe avocados, peeled and pitted
Salt and freshly ground black pepper

Mix the tomatoes, onion, chili, lime juice and cilantro into a coarse paste using a food-processor or pestle and mortar.

Mash the avocados with a fork until fairly smooth, but still with some texture.

Combine the processed paste with the avocado and season to taste with salt and pepper.

If you prefer a more textured guacamole, chop the tomatoes by hand and stir into the avocado with the spiced paste.

Chosen as a source of: vitamins B6, C, E, MUFA, polyphenols / Per serving (based on 4 servings): 189 kcal; 17.8g fat; 3.7g saturated fat / 1.5 portions of fruit/vegetables

red pepper hummus

The addition of marinated red peppers adds a deep color and flavor to this hummus. It uses mostly pantry ingredients and keeps covered in the refrigerator for a few days.

SERVES 6–8

2 tablespoons tahini
2 tablespoons lemon juice
14-ounce can chickpeas, drained
2 red pepper halves, marinated in olive oil

1 large garlic clove, grated or crushed
2 tablespoons olive oil
Pinch of paprika
Pinch of cumin
Salt

Place the tahini and the lemon juice in a food-processor and pulse for a minute.

Add the chickpeas, peppers, garlic, olive oil, spices and 3 tablespoons water and process for a good few minutes until smooth. Taste and adjust the seasoning, adding more lemon juice or spices if needed. If you prefer a looser texture, add some more water.

Simply leave out the red pepper to make a standard hummus (you may need to add a little more water as you won't have the added moisture of the pepper), or replace the red pepper with marinated sun-dried tomatoes.

Chosen as a source of: vitamin C, pulses, polyphenols / Per serving (based on 6 servings): 129 kcal; 9g fat; 1.3g saturated fat / 0.5 portions of fruit/vegetables

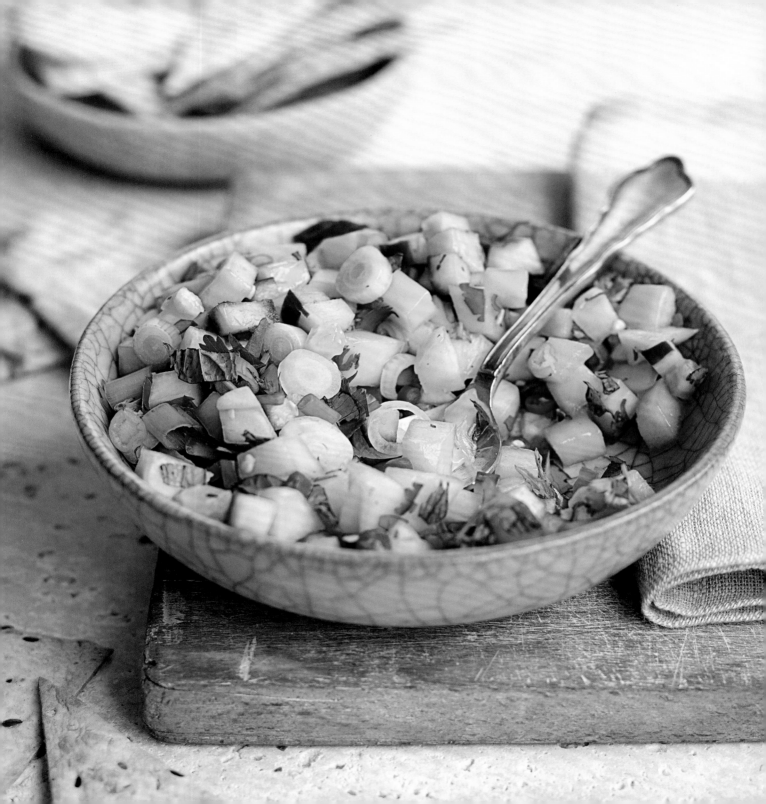

mango salsa

This vibrant salsa is refreshing with a hint of heat. It works well as an accompaniment to fish dishes or can be chopped more finely and served as a dip. This can be prepared ahead of time, which will also allow the flavors to develop.

SERVES 2 AS A SIDE OR 4–6 AS A DIP

1 mango, peeled and pitted
2-inch piece of cucumber (about 1¾ ounces)
1 scallion, finely chopped
1 tablespoon finely chopped fresh mint
1 tablespoon finely chopped cilantro
½ small red chili, seeded if preferred, finely chopped (optional)
Juice of ½ lime

Cut the mango and cucumber into similar bite-size chunks (if using as a dip, you may want to aim for smaller chunks).

Place the mango, cucumber, scallion, mint, cilantro and chili into a bowl. Add the lime juice and gently combine all the ingredients. Keep in the refrigerator until needed.

Chosen as a source of: vitamin C, polyphenols / Per serving (based on 2 servings): 75 kcal; 0.4g fat; 0.1g saturated fat / 1.5 portions of fruit/vegetables

tomato and pepper salsa

There are lots of variations on a tomato salsa. A basic tomato salsa will contain tomatoes, onion, some acidic liquid like lime or lemon juice and some fresh herbs. This one includes red pepper too, but go ahead and experiment with different variations on the theme.

SERVES 4–6

3 ripe tomatoes, cubed
1 roasted red pepper, marinated in olive oil, chopped
1 scallion, finely chopped
½ small red chili, seeded if preferred, finely chopped (optional)
2 tablespoons finely chopped cilantro
Juice of ½ lime
Small pinch of salt

Place the tomatoes, pepper, scallion, chili and cilantro in a bowl and stir to combine.

Add the lime juice and salt and stir through.

Taste and adjust the seasoning, adding more lime juice and/or chili if needed.

Try using red onion instead of the scallions or parsley instead of the cilantro. Add a bit of garlic if you are leaving out the chili. You could also add some cucumber or chopped avocado.

Chosen as a source of: vitamin C, polyphenols / Per serving (based on 4 servings): 26 kcal; 0.4g fat; 0.1g saturated fat / 1.5 portions of fruit/vegetables

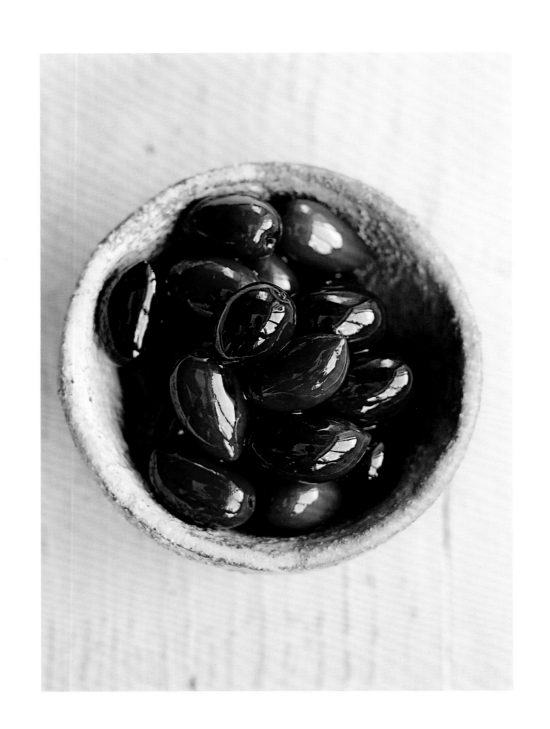

tapenade

Tapenade has a strong, deep flavor and is fairly high in salt so is usually used in small quantities. It can be used as a topping for fish or chicken, added to casseroles or spread on crusty bread. It will keep covered in the refrigerator for a few days.

SERVES 4–6

7 ounces (about 1¾ cups) good-quality black olives, pitted
1 tablespoon capers
3 anchovy fillets
1 small garlic clove, finely chopped or crushed
2 tablespoons olive oil
1 tablespoon lemon juice
1 teaspoon Dijon mustard
½ teaspoon dried thyme
1 tablespoon freshly chopped flat-leaf parsley

Put the pitted olives, capers, anchovies and garlic into a food-processor and blend briefly. (If you don't have a food-processor, you can use a pestle and mortar instead.)

Add the olive oil, lemon juice, mustard and herbs and continue processing or grinding until it forms a rough paste.

Chosen as a source of: MUFA, fish/seafood, polyphenols / Per serving (based on 4 servings): 184 kcal; 18.5g fat; 2.3g saturated fat / 0.5 portion of fruit/vegetables

tasty tomato sauce

This delicious savory-sweet sauce has a much deeper flavor than most sauces you can buy and has no unwanted additives. It is really easy to make, keeps well in the refrigerator for several days or can be frozen for up to four months.

SERVES 4

1 tablespoon canola oil
1 large onion, finely chopped
2–3 garlic cloves, finely chopped
2 x 14-ounce cans plum tomatoes
2 bay leaves
2–3 canned anchovy fillets, drained and finely chopped
1 teaspoon good-quality balsamic vinegar
Salt and freshly ground black pepper

Heat the canola oil in a large pan over medium heat. Add the onions and garlic and cook gently until softened.

Add the tomatoes, bay leaves and anchovy fillets to the pan and stir well. Bring to a boil, then reduce the heat and simmer gently, uncovered, for 20–30 minutes, stirring occasionally to break up the tomatoes, until the sauce is thick and pulpy.

Stir in the balsamic vinegar and plenty of ground black pepper. Taste before adding salt as the anchovies add some saltiness.

This sauce can be stirred through pasta for a simple supper or used as the basis for a wide range of dishes, including many from this book such as Tortilla Pizza (page 59), Eggplant and Tomato Gratin (page 56), Sea Bream Provençale (page 105), Eggplant Pasticcio (page 123) and Roasted Mediterranean Butternut Squash (page 120).

The addition of anchovies means this sauce is not suitable for strict vegetarians, so leave them out and add an extra teaspoon of balsamic vinegar if cooking for vegetarians.

Chosen as a source of: vitamins B6, C, E, folate, fish/seafood, polyphenols / Per serving: 89 kcal; 3.7g fat; 0.2g saturated fat / 3 portions of fruit/vegetables

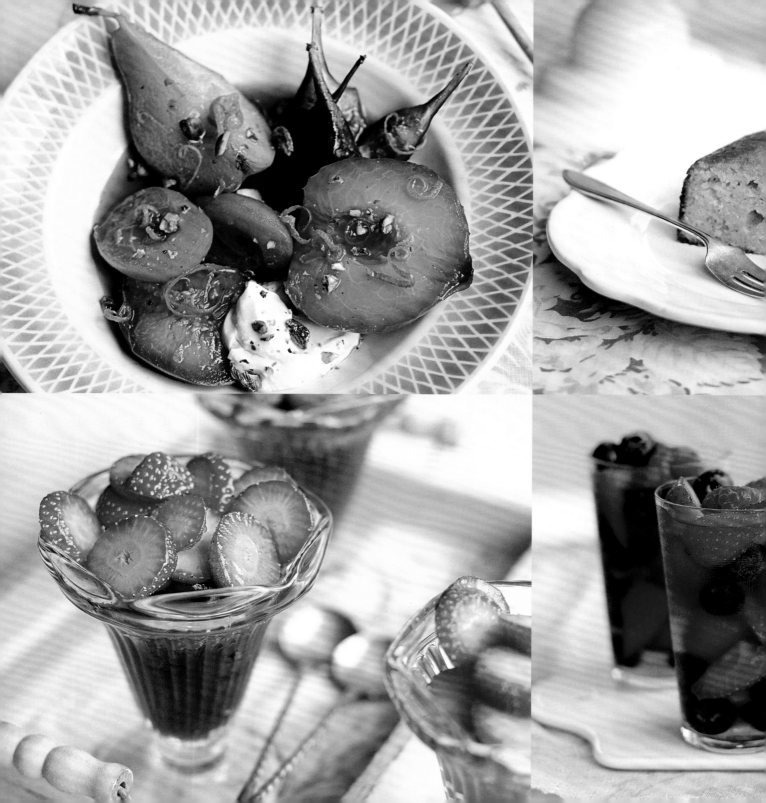

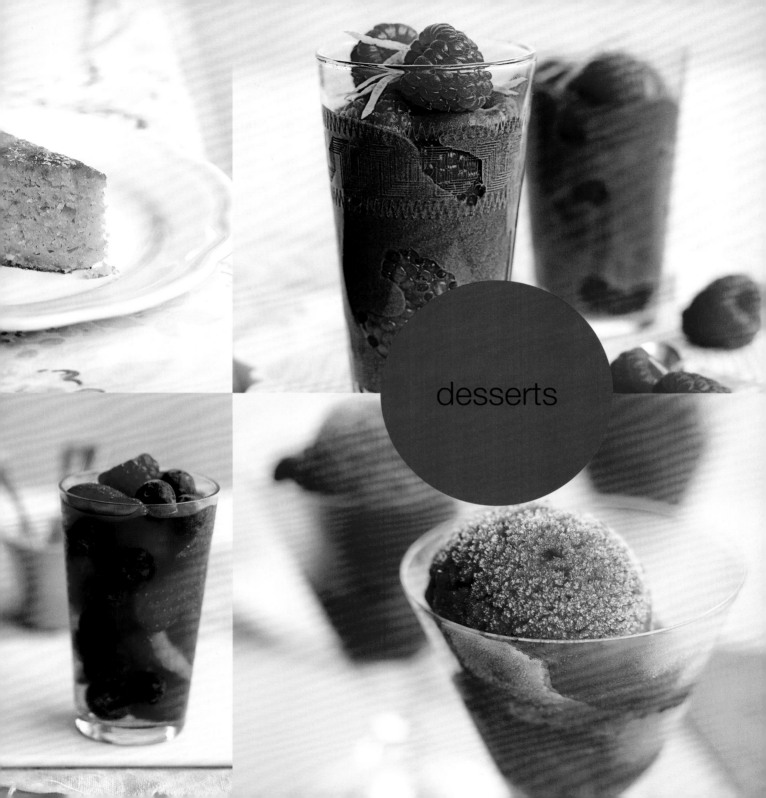

desserts

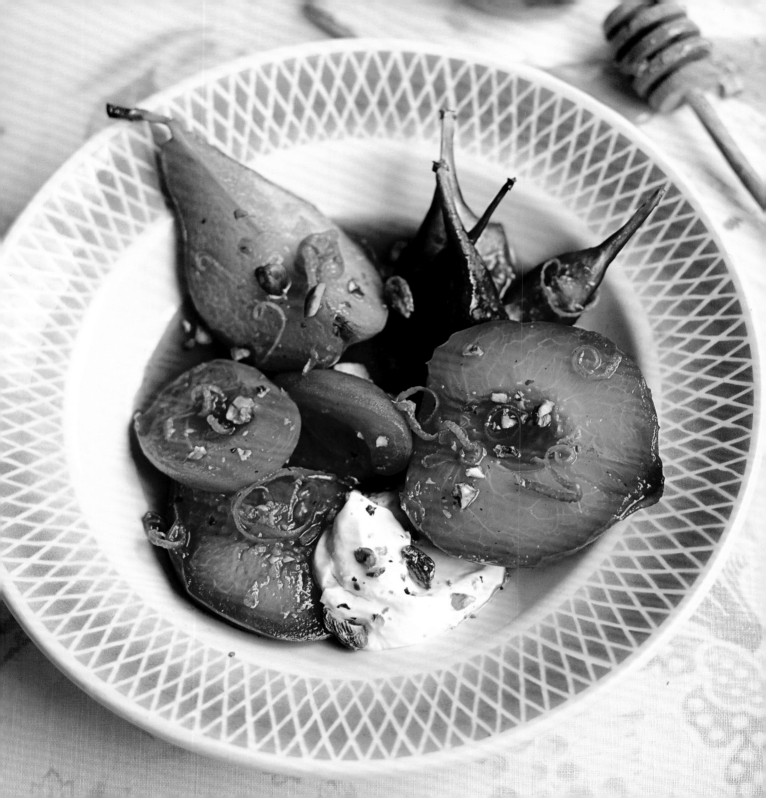

baked fruit with nuts and honey

A wonderfully different way to enjoy fruit and great for when you want something sweet and warming.

SERVES 4

2 pears
4 fresh figs
2 peaches or nectarines
2 plums or apricots
1 tablespoon brown sugar
Juice of 2 oranges
Zest of 1 orange

10½ ounces (scant 1½ cups) nonfat yogurt
1 tablespoon honey, plus extra to drizzle (optional)
2 handfuls of unsalted shelled pistachios, roughly chopped

Preheat the oven to 350°F.

Wash the fruits. Quarter the pears and remove the cores. Cut a cross on the top of the figs and set aside. Pit and halve the remaining fruits.

Place all the fruits (except the figs) cut-side down on a baking sheet.

Mix the sugar and orange juice and zest together and pour over the fruits. Bake for 10 minutes, then add the figs and bake for another 15 minutes or until the fruits are soft and caramelized on the bottom (this will depend on how ripe they were to start with).

Meanwhile, mix the yogurt and honey together in a serving bowl. Remove the fruit from the oven and serve with a dollop of yogurt and a sprinkle of pistachios. Drizzle over a little more honey, if required.

Any combination of fruits can be used. Choose seasonal, ripe fruits and simply adjust the cooking time by reducing it for smaller, softer, riper fruits. Aim to choose different colors—this will improve the look of the dish and may maximize the range of nutrients.

Chosen as a source of: vitamin C / Per serving: 262 kcal; 8.7g fat; 1.2g saturated fat / 3 portions of fruit/vegetables

baked stuffed apples

This recipe is adapted from a favorite Sunday dessert and produces its own tasty syrup while baking. Delicious served with low-fat custard or nonfat Greek yogurt.

SERVES 4

4 medium cooking apples
5½ ounces (about 1 cup) pitted dates, chopped
1¾ ounces (about ½ cup) chopped nuts (Brazils, pistachios or almonds, or combination of all)

Finely grated zest and juice of 1 large orange
¼ cup demerara sugar
Scant ⅔ cup water

Preheat the oven to 350°F.

Wash and dry the apples. Do not peel but remove the stem and core with an apple corer or a thin, sharp knife. You should be left with a whole apple with a cylindrical hole in the middle. Score a line around the circumference of the widest part of the apple with a sharp knife. This will prevent the apples from splitting as the flesh expands when they cook.

Mix together the dates, chopped nuts and orange zest. Place the apples in a shallow baking dish, divide the stuffing mixture into four and use to fill the hole in the center of each apple. Press the filling down firmly so that each hole is completely filled.

Drizzle the orange juice over the apples and sprinkle the demerara sugar on top. Pour the water into the base of the dish, cover it with foil and bake in the preheated oven for 45–60 minutes until the apples are completely tender. You can test this by piercing from the side with a sharp knife or skewer.

Serve warm or cold—this dish reheats very well.

If you are not a fan of dates, dried figs or apricots also work well in this recipe.

Chosen as a source of: vitamins C, E, polyphenols / Per serving: 282 kcal; 7.6g fat; 0.9g saturated fat / 2 portions of fruit/vegetables

mulled fruits

A delicious, warming way to enjoy fruit. This would make a lovely alternative to Christmas pudding, either on its own or served with the Spiced Clementine Cake on page 153.

SERVES 4

½ cup red wine
3½ tablespoons orange juice
¼ cup soft brown sugar
6 cloves, 1 bay leaf and 1 cinnamon stick, or 1 packet of mulling spices
2 teaspoons arrowroot
9 ounces ripe purple plums, pitted and thickly sliced
9 ounces blackberries
5½ ounces raspberries

Place the wine, orange juice, sugar and spices in a pan. Heat gently until the sugar has dissolved, then bring to a boil and simmer for about 5 minutes. Remove and discard the spices.

Mix the arrowroot with a splash of water and mix to make a thin paste. Stir into the spiced wine and continue stirring over medium heat until thickened.

Add the plums and blackberries to the pan and simmer for 2–3 minutes. Stir in the raspberries. Taste for sweetness and add a little more sugar if the fruit is too tart.

Serve hot, cold or at room temperature.

Other fruits such as pears, peaches, nectarines and strawberries will also work in this recipe but cooking times may need to be adjusted.

Chosen as a source of: vitamins C, E, folate, polyphenols / Per serving: 130 kcal; 0.4g fat; 0.1g saturated fat / 2 portions of fruit/vegetables

chocolate and orange mousse

This rich-tasting recipe allows you to indulge yourself. It has been kindly provided by Gino D'Acampo.

SERVES 6

7 ounces good-quality bittersweet chocolate, chopped
4 free-range eggs
Zest and juice of 1 orange
11¼ ounces raspberries

Melt the chocolate in a heatproof bowl over a pan of simmering water, making sure that the base of the bowl does not touch the water. Set aside to cool, but don't let it harden again.

Meanwhile, separate the eggs into two clean, dry bowls. Whisk the egg whites until stiff peaks form.

Beat the egg yolks together with the orange juice and half the zest for 2 minutes. With a metal spoon, gently fold the melted chocolate into the egg yolk mixture a little at a time. Lastly, fold in the egg whites until all the ingredients are combined.

Divide the raspberries between six dessert glasses, each holding about 1 scant cup. Pour the chocolate mixture over the raspberries and cover with plastic wrap. Leave to rest in the refrigerator for 3 hours until set.

Just before serving, remove the plastic wrap and decorate with the remaining orange zest.

This recipe contains uncooked eggs and is best avoided by pregnant women and the very elderly.

Chosen as a source of: vitamins B12, C, folate, polyphenols / Per serving: 237 kcal; 13.1g fat; 6.6g saturated fat / 0.5 portion of fruit/vegetables

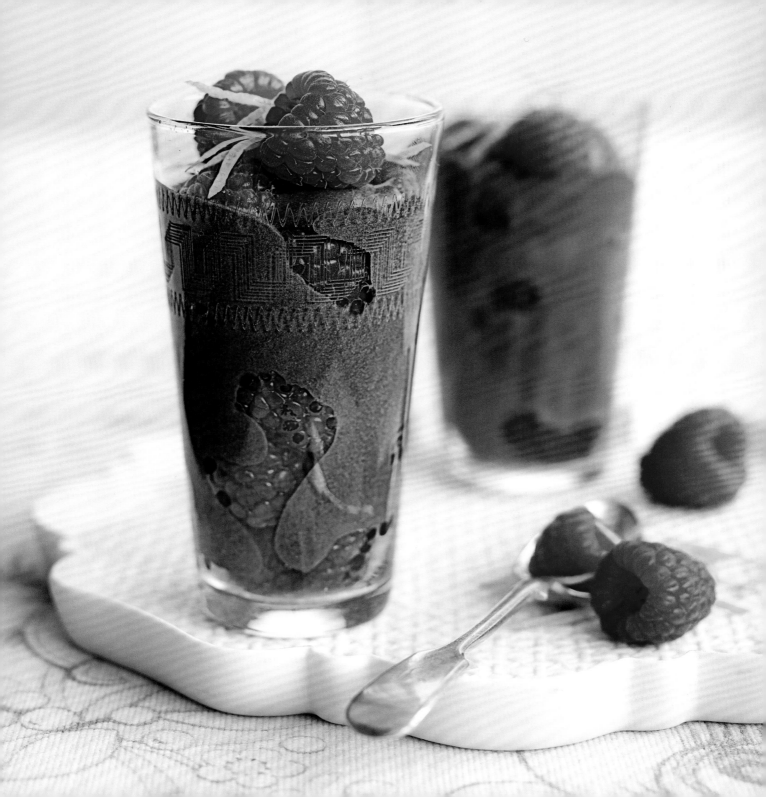

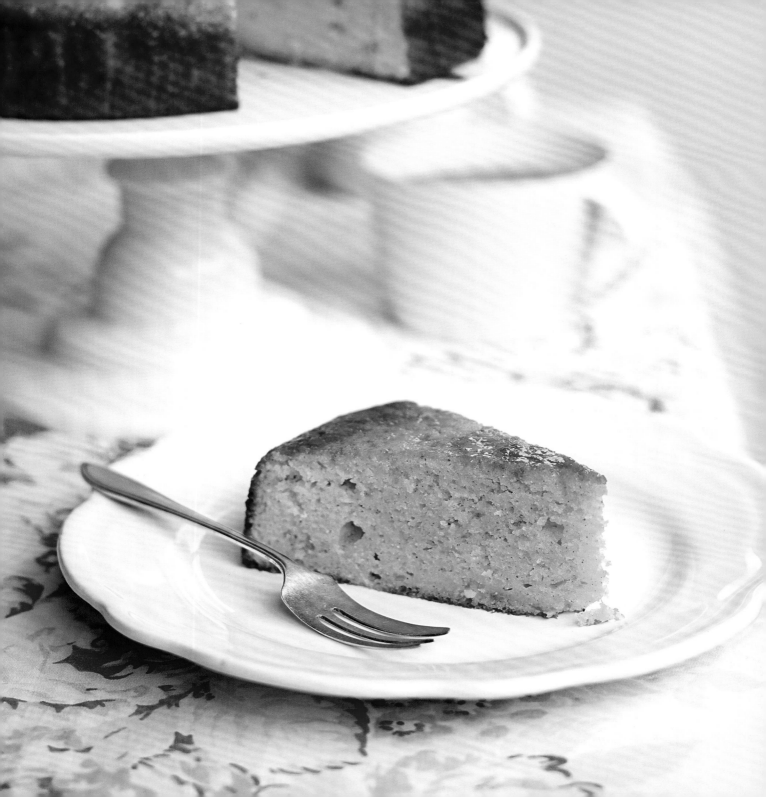

spiced clementine cake

A feisty cake, rich with citrus and spices.

SERVES 12

For the cake
4–5 whole clementines (about 12 ounces in total), unpeeled
6 tablespoons all-purpose flour
1 teaspoon baking powder
1 cup superfine sugar
2½ cups ground almonds
1 teaspoon cardamom seeds (from about 15–20 green cardamom pods), ground

¼ teaspoon ground cinnamon
6 free-range eggs, lightly beaten
Seeds from 1 vanilla bean or 1 teaspoon vanilla extract

For the glaze
Juice of ½ pink grapefruit
1½ tablespoons superfine sugar

Place the clementines in a pan and just cover with water. Bring to a boil, cover, and simmer gently for 1½–2 hours until very soft. Drain the fruit and leave until cool enough to handle.

Preheat the oven to 325°F. Lightly oil and line a 9-inch springform cake pan with parchment paper.

Cut each clementine in half and discard the pips. Blend the fruit, including the skin, in a food-processor into a smooth pulp.

Sift the flour and baking powder into a large mixing bowl. Stir in the sugar, ground almonds, ground cardamom seeds and cinnamon. Make a well in the center and add the eggs, clementine pulp and vanilla seeds or extract. Mix well. Pour into the lined pan and bake on the middle shelf of the oven for 40–60 minutes. Check after 40 minutes and cover with foil if it is getting too brown. The cake is ready when a skewer inserted into the center comes out clean.

Just before the cake is due to come out of the oven, heat the grapefruit juice and sugar in a small pan, stirring, until the sugar dissolves. Bring to a boil and simmer for 2–3 minutes.

Remove the cake from the oven, leave it in the pan and pierce the top with a cocktail stick in several places. Drizzle the pink grapefruit glaze over the cake, making sure it covers the whole of the top of the cake. Leave to cool in the pan for 20 minutes, then remove from the cake pan and serve warm or transfer to a wire rack to cool completely.

For Spiced Lemon Cake: Replace the clementines with 3 thin-skinned lemons and the cardamom and cinnamon with 1 teaspoon of chopped fresh thyme leaves and 1 teaspoon of caraway seeds that have been bruised in a pestle and mortar. A clementine glaze made with the juice of 2 clementines and 4 teaspoons of superfine sugar works well on the lemon cake.

Chosen as a source of: vitamins B12, C, E, MUFA, polyphenols / Per serving: 265 kcal; 13.7g fat; 1.6g saturated fat / 0.5 portions of fruit/vegetables

chestnut and chocolate cake

Thank you to Gino D'Acampo for this recipe, originally published in his book *The Italian Diet*. This cake is made with no added fat and is delicious warm or cold.

SERVES 16

Vegetable oil, for greasing
1¾ cups + 2 tablespoons all-purpose flour
1¼ cups good-quality cocoa powder, plus extra for dusting
1 teaspoon baking powder
2 teaspoons baking soda
1 cup superfine sugar
Pinch of salt

2 teaspoons vanilla extract
9¼ ounces chestnut puree
2 large free-range eggs
1 cup skim milk
1 cup cold strong coffee, preferably espresso (or made with 3 heaped teaspoons instant coffee)

Preheat the oven to 350°F. Lightly grease and line an 8½-inch springform cake pan.

Sift the flour, cocoa powder, baking powder and baking soda into a large bowl. Add the sugar, salt, vanilla extract, chestnut puree and eggs. Pour in the milk and mix until well combined. Add the coffee and mix well.

Pour the mixture into the cake pan and bake in the middle of the oven for about 45 minutes. The cake is cooked when a skewer inserted into the center comes out clean. Leave the cake to cool in the pan for 5 minutes, then turn out onto a large serving plate and dust with cocoa powder.

Chosen as a source of: polyphenols / Per serving: 172 kcal; 3.4g fat; 1.3g saturated fat

velvet cocoa sauce

This thick, smooth, cocoa-rich, bitter chocolate sauce provides a delicious contrast of flavor when served with sweet fruits or desserts.

SERVES 2–4

½ cup good-quality cocoa powder
Scant ½ cup water

3 tablespoons maple syrup
1 tablespoon low-fat thick cream

Place the cocoa powder and water in a small pan and heat gently, stirring, until the mixture begins to thicken.

Add the maple syrup and simmer gently for 1–2 minutes.

Stir in the cream. Check the sweetness is to your taste, adding a little more maple syrup if required. Serve hot or cold to accompany sweet desserts. Any leftover sauce reheats well.

If you prefer a thinner sauce, simply add a little more water.

Chosen as a source of: polyphenols / Per serving (based on 2 servings): 155 kcal; 6.5g fat; 3.9g saturated fat

avocado, chocolate and strawberry dessert

At last, an indulgent, chocolaty dessert that's actually good for you! This creamy dessert is refreshing and much less sweet than many other chocolate puddings. It is best made and served on the same day.

SERVES 6

9 ounces fresh strawberries
1 tablespoon powdered sugar
3 very ripe avocados
½ cup good-quality cocoa powder

6½ tablespoons maple syrup
3½ tablespoons water
Seeds from 1 vanilla bean

Hull the strawberries, slice thickly and arrange them in a single layer in a shallow dish. Sprinkle over the powdered sugar, cover with plastic wrap and leave in a cool place for an hour until the strawberries have softened slightly and released some of their juice.

Cut the avocados in half, carefully remove the pits and scoop out the flesh with a spoon. Don't worry if some of the flesh is turning brown—this is a sign of ripeness and won't be evident once the cocoa has been added.

Place the avocado flesh, cocoa powder, maple syrup, water and vanilla seeds in a food-processor and blend until smooth. You may need to scrape down the sides of the bowl a couple of times.

Once the mixture is completely smooth, divide it between six dessert bowls or sundae glasses and top with the strawberries and their juice. Serve immediately.

Raspberries or a mixed berry compote would also work well with the chocolate cream.

Chosen as a source of: vitamins B6, C, E, MUFA, polyphenols / Per serving: 387 kcal; 29g fat; 7.1g saturated fat / 2.5 portions of fruit/vegetables

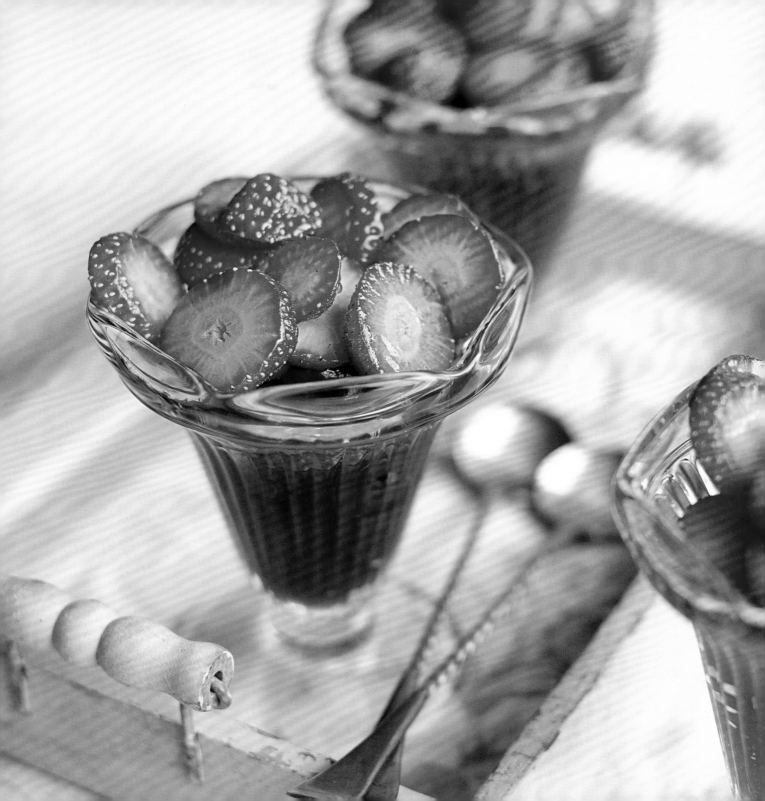

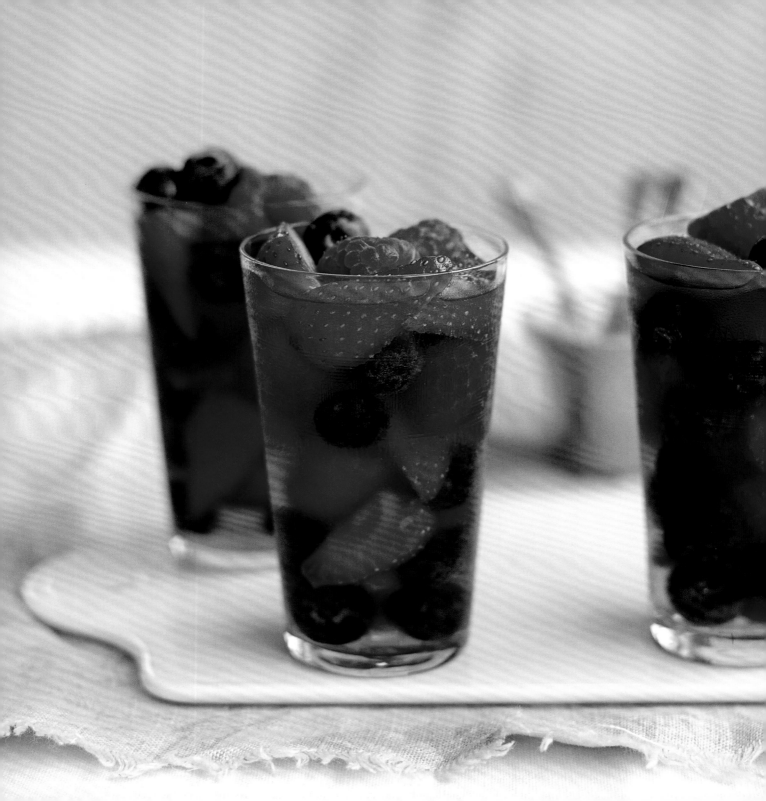

summer fruit jello

A pretty dessert that works equally well at a relaxed summer lunch or a more formal dinner.

SERVES 4

2½ sheets leaf gelatin
Generous 1½ cups sparkling
   rosé wine
5 tablespoons superfine sugar

11¼ ounces mixed summer
   fruits (blueberries, raspberries,
   strawberries)

Put the gelatin sheets in a bowl of cold water to soften.

Heat the rosé in a small pan and bring to a boil. Add the sugar and stir until dissolved. Remove from the heat.

Remove the gelatin from the water and squeeze out the liquid. Add to the wine mixture and stir until completely dissolved. Transfer to a jug and leave to cool until tepid.

While the jello mix is cooling, divide the berries between four individual serving glasses. If the strawberries are very large, cut them into smaller pieces.

When the jello mixture is cool (but not cold) pour over the fruit in the glasses. The tips of the fruit may not be completely covered but this is fine. Put in the refrigerator to set for several hours or overnight.

You can replace the gelatin with a reduced-sugar jello (e.g. raspberry), made up with 1 cup of the rosé. When cool, add the rest of the wine—this helps retain the bubbles. Substitute white grape juice for the wine if you are making this for children or prefer not to use alcohol.

Chosen as a source of: vitamin C, polyphenols / Per serving: 157 kcal; 0.1g fat; 0g saturated fat / 1 portion of fruit/vegetables

vibrant fruit salad

Fruit salads are really only limited by your imagination. Most combinations of fruit work and using fruits that are in season will ensure the best flavor. Cut them into bite-size cubes and serve in a bowl, slice and arrange on a platter, or make fruit skewers for a bit of fun. The added mint is optional—some people say it makes the salad, while others are not so keen.

SERVES 4

1 mango, peeled and pitted
½ small watermelon
   (about 10½ ounces)
2 kiwis, peeled
20 black grapes

1 passion fruit
5–10 mint leaves (optional)
2 tablespoons orange juice
1 tablespoon lemon juice

Cut the mango, watermelon and kiwis into ¾-inch cubes and halve the grapes. Place the cut fruit into a salad bowl.

Cut the passion fruit in half and scoop the seeds and pulp out into the bowl. Shred the mint leaves (if using) and add to the salad.

Pour the orange juice and lemon juice over the fruit and stir to combine and coat all the ingredients. Cover with plastic wrap and let it rest for 30 minutes to let all the flavors combine.

Be sure to give it a stir before serving to coat the fruits in the lovely juice.

By including a range of different colors, you will maximize the nutrients you get—so go ahead and "eat a rainbow."

Chosen as a source of: vitamins B6, C, polyphenols / Per serving: 97 kcal; 0.6g fat; 0.2g saturated fat / 2.5 portions of fruit/vegetables

mango and lime sorbet

The addition of the rum gives the sorbet a taste of the Caribbean, as well as ensuring it doesn't set too hard. This is a very light-tasting sorbet that isn't too sweet.

SERVES 4

1 pound fresh or frozen mango
2 tablespoons rum
3 tablespoons superfine sugar, or to taste
4 tablespoons water
Juice of ½ small lime

If you are using frozen mango, you may need to let it defrost a bit in order to blend easily.

Place all the ingredients in blender and blend until smooth. Taste and add more sugar if needed, bearing in mind that some of the sweetness will be reduced once frozen.

If you have an ice-cream machine, process according to the manufacturer's instructions. Alternatively, pour the mixture into a freezerproof container and place in the freezer. After an hour, remove and break up the ice crystals using a fork. Return to the freezer and repeat until the sorbet is frozen.

The sorbet can be served immediately or transferred to a rigid container and frozen until required. It will keep well in the freezer for several weeks, although you will need to transfer from freezer to refrigerator to soften for a few minutes before serving.

For a summer fruit alternative, use about a pound of summer berries, add 2 tablespoons of cherry liqueur and leave out the lime. If you use fruits with small seeds, such as raspberries or strawberries, strain the fruit puree before freezing.

Chosen as a source of: vitamin C, polyphenols / Per serving: 119 kcal; 0.2g fat; 0.1g saturated fat / 1.5 portions of fruit/vegetables

cranberry sorbet

This yummy sorbet has a really creamy mouthfeel and makes a luscious accompaniment to fruit salad or chocolate-dipped fruit.

SERVES 6

1 pound 2 ounces fresh or frozen cranberries
1½ cups superfine sugar
Generous 2 cups water

Place the berries in a pan with the sugar and water. Bring to a boil, stirring occasionally, then cover and simmer on gentle heat for about 15 minutes or until the berries have popped out of their skins and are soft.

Carefully pour the mixture into a blender or food-processor and puree until it looks almost completely smooth. Strain the mixture through a sieve to remove any bits of skin or seeds, pressing down well so as not to waste any puree. Discard the solids.

Leave the mixture to cool to room temperature, then cover and put in the refrigerator for several hours or overnight to chill.

Transfer to an ice-cream maker and process according to the manufacturer's instructions. Alternatively, pour the mixture into a freezerproof container and place in the freezer. After an hour, remove from the freezer and break up the ice crystals using a fork. Return to the freezer and repeat until the sorbet is frozen.

The sorbet can be served immediately or transferred to a rigid container and frozen until required. It will keep well in the freezer for several weeks, although you will need to transfer from freezer to refrigerator to soften for a few minutes before serving.

Chosen as a source of: vitamin C, polyphenols / Per serving: 242 kcal; 0.1g fat; 0g saturated fat / 1 portion of fruit/vegetables

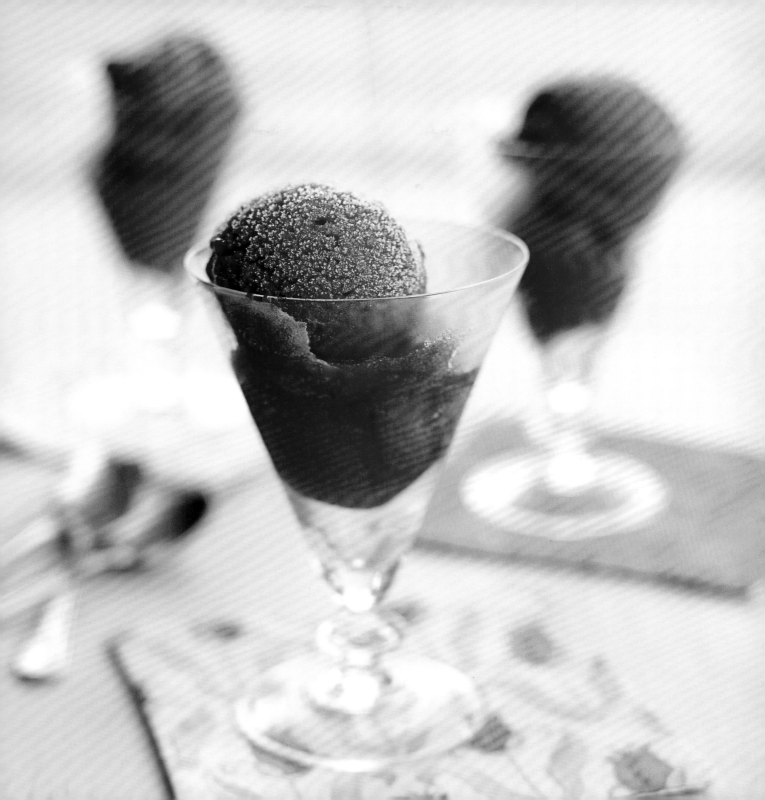

coffee and hazelnut meringues

This is an adaptation of a foolproof recipe from Vanessa's wonderful mom, Shirley Goddard— perfect served with fresh fruit for that sweet treat.

MAKES ABOUT 16 MERINGUES

3 free-range egg whites (about 4¼ ounces)
1 tablespoon white vinegar
1 cup superfine sugar
1 teaspoon baking powder

1 heaped teaspoon finely ground instant coffee powder (preferably espresso)
¾ ounce (about 2 tablespoons) hazelnuts, roughly chopped

Preheat the oven to 225°F and line a baking sheet with parchment paper.

Whisk the egg whites with the vinegar in a clean, dry bowl until soft peaks form. Continue whisking while adding the sugar slowly, a tablespoonful at a time, until all the sugar is incorporated and the mixture is glossy and forms stiff peaks.

Add the baking powder and coffee powder and whisk briefly to incorporate. Gently fold in half the chopped nuts.

Use 2 tablespoons to scoop out the mixture and shape the meringues onto the baking sheet. (Alternatively, use a piping bag for a more consistent and controlled shape.) Sprinkle the remaining nuts over the top and then bake in the oven for 1½ hours. Remove from the oven to cool—or, if a drier texture is preferred, leave the meringues in the turned-off oven to cool.

Chosen as a source of polyphenols / Per serving (based on 2 meringues per serving): 122 kcal; 1.6g fat; 0.1g saturated fat

Glossary

Acetylcholine. A chemical messenger involved in mental processes. Alzheimer's disease (AD) destroys the cells that produce acetylcholine. Cholinesterase inhibitors, which increase levels of acetylcholine, can help slow progress in the early stages of the disease.

Amyloid-beta (Aβ). The protein that makes up the "amyloid plaques" that form in the brain in Alzheimer's disease and are toxic to nerve cells.

Atherosclerosis. The deposit of fats, cholesterol, calcium and other substances in the arteries to form "plaque" (not to be confused with amyloid plaques). As it accumulates, it can restrict blood flow, making it difficult for oxygen to reach the brain—a key factor in vascular dementia.

Brain atrophy. The loss or shrinkage of brain cells, which causes the brain to decrease in volume—a characteristic of many neurodegenerative diseases including Alzheimer's disease.

Cognition. The mental processes involved in learning and understanding—including thinking, remembering, perceiving, problem-solving, planning, imagining and the use of language.

Cognitive decline. Loss of the processes involved in cognition manifested in, for example, difficulties learning new things, speed of processing information, language and other cognitive processes.

Crohn's disease. A chronic inflammatory bowel disease.

DNA. Deoxyribonucleic acid—the famous "double helix" molecule that carries genetic information needed for the development and function of living organisms.

Endothelium. The thin layer of cells that lines the inner surface of blood vessels, the cavities of the heart and the vessels that carry lymph around the body. Endothelial dysfunction can be induced by oxidative stress and may be involved in both vascular dementia and Alzheimer's disease.

Executive function. The mental processes involved in linking past and present experience—for example keeping track of time, managing attention, switching tasks, planning, organizing, remembering detail, curbing inappropriate speech or behavior.

Loss of executive function is a feature of cognitive decline and dementia.

Gene. A section of DNA that provides the instructions for making a particular protein. The ApoE gene provides the instructions for making the protein apolipoprotein E (ApoE), which carries cholesterol and other fats through the bloodstream.

Gene variant. A version of a gene. The ApoE gene has at least three variants. The ApoE ε4 variant is linked to increased risk of Alzheimer's disease, while the ApoE ε2 variant is thought to be protective.

Hippocampus. A region of the brain concerned with memory formation and retrieval. Atrophy of the hippocampus is a feature of Alzheimer's disease and may also occur in vascular dementia.

Hormone. A chemical messenger produced in one part of the body that regulates the activity of cells or organs in other parts.

Insulin. A hormone produced by the pancreas that is responsible for moving glucose from the bloodstream into the muscles and other tissues.

Insulin resistance. A state in which the body's cells are unable to respond to insulin. Linked with obesity, type-2 diabetes and non-alcoholic fatty-liver disease, there is increasing evidence that it may be involved in the development of Alzheimer's disease.

Marker. A substance in the blood or other cells or tissues that can highlight the presence of disease. The identification of reliable blood markers for Alzheimer's disease would make it much easier to diagnose, enabling people with it to get early help.

Megaloblastic anemia. A blood disorder caused by a deficiency of folic acid or vitamin B12 and marked by the appearance of very large red blood cells.

Neurodegenerative diseases. Conditions involving the degeneration and/or death of neurons in the brain—including Parkinson's, Alzheimer's and Huntington's diseases.

Neurofibrillary tangles. Twisted masses of a protein called tau found in the brains of people with Alzheimer's disease.

Neurons. Nerve cells found in the brain and spinal cord.

Neurotransmitter. A messenger chemical produced by nerve cells.

Non-melanoma skin cancer. A type of skin cancer.

Noradrenaline (norepinephrine). The body's "fight-or-flight" hormone, which helps to keep us alert and retain what we have learned. It is reduced in Alzheimer's disease.

Osteomalacia. Softening and weakening of the bones in adults, often caused by vitamin D deficiency.

Pernicious anemia. A condition in which the body can't make enough healthy red blood cells due to vitamin B12 deficiency.

Processing speed. The speed at which we can accomplish simple cognitive tasks demanding attention and focused concentration. It is used as a measure of cognitive function.

Reactive oxygen species (ROS). Unstable molecules formed as part of normal metabolism that include oxygen free radicals. They perform important functions in cells but at high levels can be damaging. Polyunsaturated fatty acids are especially susceptible to ROS damage.

Rickets. Softening and weakening of bones in children, usually due to severe, prolonged vitamin D deficiency.

Selenoproteins. A small class of proteins that contain selenium and carry out actions, such as combating oxidative stress and reducing inflammation. They play a crucial role in brain function.

Visual memory. The part of the memory we use to understand what we see.

Working memory. The part of the memory we use to hold information in the mind so we can perform a cognitive task.

Appendix 1:
Exercise and dementia

A healthy diet is only one part of the equation for a healthy brain. Numerous studies show that regular physical exercise benefits health—stronger bones, healthier heart, lungs and joints—as well as protecting against conditions such as cancer, diabetes and heart disease. It is also becoming clear that it is vital for a healthy brain. Regular exercise is linked to a lower risk of dementia and AD—and there are indications that it may help improve cognitive function in people with mild cognitive impairment (MCI). There is also exciting research emerging showing that exercise and nutrition have a synergistic effect.

What activities are the most beneficial?

Having a strong heart and lungs (cardiorespiratory fitness) has been linked to better cognitive function in several studies dating from the late 1980s. These show that fitter older people do better in tests of mental performance than their inactive peers. Other studies that have followed people up over several years and a number of RCTs support this finding. Aerobic exercise contributes to heart and lung strength.

Recent research has shown that, perhaps surprisingly, resistance or strength training may also benefit the brain. This type of exercise seems to improve cognitive function, including both short and long-term memory, attention and decision-making skills.

How often should you do them?

The earlier in life you start exercising the better, according to researchers from King's College London. Regular intensive lifelong activity is likely to achieve the best results but even exercising less often and less intensively could have benefits, they say. But it is not too late, even if you leave it until midlife to start to move more. A US study found that people who were the fittest in middle age had a lower risk of developing dementia of any kind later on.

What effect can exercise have?

Exercise may help protect against dementia in several ways including:

- improving heart health and increasing blood flow to the brain
- affecting hormones by increasing levels of estrogen and testosterone, which may be neuroprotective; some scientists think that exercise may lower levels of the hormone insulin, which is increasingly thought to play a role in dementia
- boosting immunity
- helping to improve metabolism
- encouraging formation of new nerve cells (neurogenesis) in the brain
- promoting the formation of new connections between nerve cells (synaptogenesis) and offshoots from existing blood vessels in the brain (angiogenesis)
- encouraging production of "growth factors," vital for keeping the brain healthy
- enhancing the effects of a healthy diet—people who exercise regularly are more likely to have other healthy habits such as eating a good diet.

Our recommendations

Although, as with nutrition research, we still have to dot a few i's and cross a few t's, the weight of evidence suggests that being physically active can help protect your brain. We recommend the following:

- Include both aerobic exercise—such as walking, jogging, swimming, dancing—and resistance (strength) exercise using free weights, machines at the gym or your own body weight.
- If you haven't been active at all or not for a while, start gently and gradually increase the intensity and frequency of the exercise you do.
- Aim to build up to the 150 minutes of exercise a week—or 30 minutes most days—recommended in many national guidelines (this is still effective if split into smaller "chunks" of 10 or 15 minutes). If this is too much, even exercising once a week will help.
- If you have health or mobility problems, consult your doctor before starting to exercise.

Appendix 2: Weighing evidence from studies

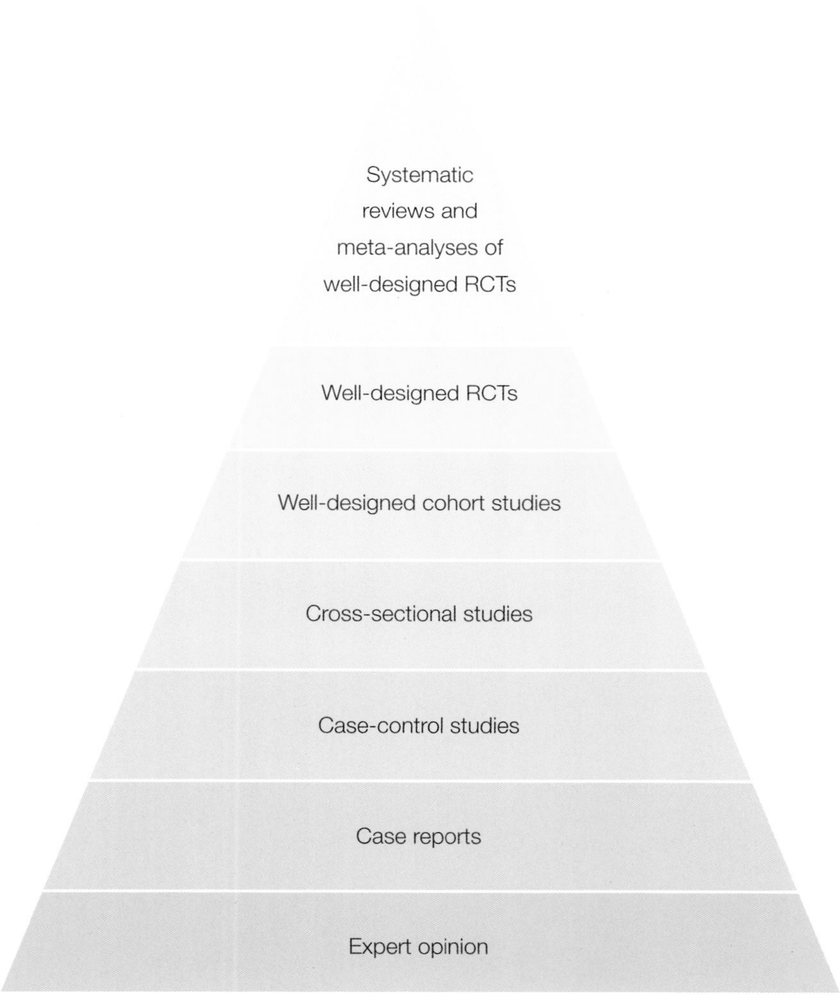

Systematic
reviews and
meta-analyses of
well-designed RCTs

Well-designed RCTs

Well-designed cohort studies

Cross-sectional studies

Case-control studies

Case reports

Expert opinion

To put this cookbook together we scoured relevant published scientific and biomedical literature to reach conclusions as to which foods and nutrients might have a positive effect on dementia, taking into account the quality of the evidence from different studies and study types.

Epidemiological studies—studies to try to determine which factors are associated with disease and which factors may protect against them—are often graded by the relative strength of their findings in a "Hierarchy of Evidence." Generally, the higher up the methods are ranked, the more robust the conclusions are assumed to be—see figure.

The quality of evidence is generally accepted as decreasing from 1 to 7.

1. **Systematic reviews and meta-analyses of well-designed randomized controlled trials (RCTs)** are organized methods of locating, assembling and evaluating the literature on a particular topic using specific criteria. A meta-analysis is a systematic review in which results from many different research studies are pooled using a statistical process to produce a more precise and reliable result.

2. **Well-designed RCTs** recruit a number of people from the same population who are randomly assigned to two (or more)

groups to test a specific treatment or, in the case of dietary research, a food or nutrient. One group receives the treatment being tested, the other (control group) receives an alternative or dummy treatment (placebo). The groups are followed up to see how effective the test treatment was.

3. **Well-designed cohort studies** are observational studies that follow groups of people (cohorts) who share common characteristics or experiences, such as their year of birth, area in which they live or occupation, over a long period. In prospective cohort studies, a group without the condition in question at the start of the study is followed for a substantial period to see who develops it. The occurrence of the condition can then be correlated with an "exposure," for example to smoking, alcohol or a food, to see if this relates to risk.

4. **Cross-sectional** studies are observational studies that involve collecting data from a population at a specific point in time, a bit like a snapshot: for example, to see whether there are fewer people with dementia who eat fish.

5. **Case-control studies** are observational studies that compare people with a disease or outcome of interest (cases) with people without (controls). Researchers look back in time to identify which people (subjects) in each group had the exposure — for example, a high intake of a beneficial food or nutrient — and compare the frequency of the exposure in the case group to the control group to pinpoint the relationship with the disease.

6. **Case reports** are detailed reports of the symptoms, signs, diagnosis, treatment and follow-up of an individual patient.

7. **Expert opinion** from expert committees, organizations or individuals; this is the lowest level of evidence.

Limitations of this system

Although widely accepted, there are several concerns about the appropriateness of the Hierarchy of Evidence. Meta-analyses, for example, which are at the top of the evidence pyramid, are secondary analyses, that is analyses of data collected for some other purpose, which means they are only as good as the studies on which they are based.

The use of evidence hierarchies has also been criticized as giving RCTs too much authority. Not all research questions can be answered through RCTs, because of either practical or ethical issues. Nutritional RCTs especially have inbuilt limitations. In the real world people can see what they are eating, meaning that it is impossible to "blind" them as to which "treatment" they are receiving. RCTs are also very expensive to perform and may often be of too short a duration to answer the research question. This is likely to be true of RCTs that try to estimate the effect of foods/nutrients on risk of dementia due to the long latency period of the disease.

RCTs that have used unsound methods do not invariably trump sound observational studies. Different types of research question are best answered by different types of study. For example, the link between smoking and lung cancer was first identified, not through RCTs, but via cohort studies carried out in the 1950s.

We recognize that the level of evidence for an effect of many foods or nutrients from individual studies may not be strong. However, an array of research evidence, all pointing to the same conclusion, from differently designed studies is the best foundation for dietary recommendations that we have at the moment. Importantly, consumption of these foods or nutrients at the level we have recommended will not be harmful and the beneficial effects may be synergistic.

Appendix 3:
Sources of beneficial foods

Sources of polyphenols

- green/black/oolong tea
- coffee
- red wine
- hard cider (traditional brew)
- cocoa/bittersweet chocolate
- berries (such as blueberries, raspberries or blackberries)
- onions
- apples
- pears
- citrus fruits
- soybeans/soy products (e.g. tofu)
- eggplant
- grapes
- apricots
- broccoli
- other fruits
- other vegetables
- legumes
- cereals
- herbs and spices

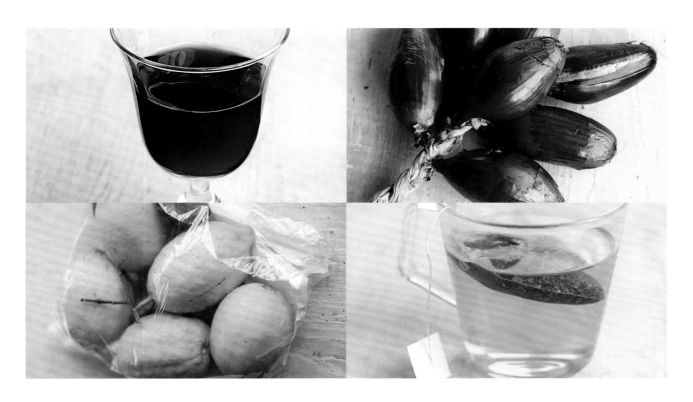

Food component	amount per 100g	portion size (g)	amount per portion
Vitamin C			
Blackcurrants	200 mg	80	160 mg
Peppers (raw)	130 mg	80 (½ pepper)	104 mg
Orange	54 mg	160 (1 medium)	86 mg
Kiwis	59 mg	60 (1 medium)	34 mg
Potatoes (new)	15 mg	150	23 mg
Cauliflower (boiled)	27 mg	80	22 mg
Tomatoes (canned)	12 mg	100	12 mg
Peas (frozen, boiled)	12 mg	80	10 mg
Apple	6 mg	100 (1 medium)	6 mg
Vitamin B6			
Fortified cereal	~1.2 mcg	40	~1.0 mcg
Chicken	0.63 mcg	130	0.8 mcg
Salmon	0.81 mcg	100	0.8 mcg
Beef	0.54 mcg	140	0.8 mcg
Mackerel, grilled	0.45 mcg	160	0.7 mcg
Veal	0.49 mcg	140	0.7 mcg
Lentils (dried)	0.93 mcg	60	0.6 mcg
Kidney	0.48 mcg	112	0.5 mcg
Herring	0.44 mcg	119	0.5 mcg
Haddock	0.41 mcg	120	0.5 mcg
Calf liver	0.63 mcg	75	0.5 mcg
Sea bream	0.46 mcg	100	0.5 mcg
Folate (Vitamin B9)			
Fortified cereals	110 mcg	40	40–140 mcg
Yeast extract	2620 mcg	10 1 tsp	262 mcg
Liver	250 mcg	100	250 mcg
Soybeans (dried)	370 mcg	60 2 tbsp	222 mcg
Orange juice	90 mcg	200 1 glass	180 mcg
Swiss chard (raw)	165 mcg	90	149 mcg
Corn	152 mcg	85	129 mcg
Black-eyed peas (boiled)	210 mcg	60 2 tbsp	126 mcg
Purple sprouting broccoli (boiled)	140 mcg	90	126 mcg

Food component	amount per 100g	portion size (g)	amount per portion
Asparagus (boiled)	83 mcg	125 5 spears	104 mcg
Brussels sprouts (boiled)	110 mcg	90	99 mcg
Beef	67 mcg	140	94 mcg
Lentils (dried)	110 mcg	80 2 tbsp	88 mcg
Kidney	70 mcg	112	78 mcg
Kidney beans (dried)	130 mcg	60 2 tbsp	78 mcg
Spinach (boiled)	81 mcg	90	73 mcg
Cabbage (raw)	75 mcg	90	68 mcg
Cauliflower (raw)	66 mcg	90	59 mcg
Chickpeas (boiled)	66 mcg	90 2 tbsp	59 mcg
Spring/collard greens (boiled)	66 mcg	90	59 mcg
Peas (raw)	62 mcg	90	56 mcg
Broccoli (boiled)	64 mcg	85 medium	54 mcg
Green/French beans (boiled)	57 mcg	90 medium	51 mcg
Beet (boiled)	110 mcg	40 average	44 mcg
Vitamin B12			
Liver	75.0 mcg	100	75 mcg
Kidney	46.0 mcg	112	52 mcg
Pilchards (canned in tomato sauce)	13.0 mcg	215 (1 small can)	28 mcg
Kipper	12.0 mcg	130	16 mcg
Mackerel	9.0 mcg	160	14 mcg
Scallops	9.0 mcg	140 (5)	13 mcg
Sardines	13.0 mcg	86 (6)	11 mcg
Mussels (without shell)	22.0 mcg	40	9 mcg
Trout	5.0 mcg	155	8 mcg
Anchovies (canned in oil)	11.0 mcg	50 (1 small can)	6 mcg
Salmon	5.0 mcg	100	5 mcg
Beef	3.0 mcg	140	4 mcg
Tuna (canned in brine)	4.0 mcg	100 (1 small can)	4 mcg
Duck	3.0 mcg	130	4 mcg
Lamb	3.0 mcg	120 (1 chop)	4 mcg

Food component	amount per 100g	portion size (g)	amount per portion
Egg yolk	6.9 mcg	36 (2 yolks)	2 mcg
Breakfast cereals	4.0 mcg	40	2 mcg
Dried seaweed	27.5 mcg	6	2 mcg
Milk	0.4 mcg	200 1 glass	1 mcg
Vitamin D			
Kipper	25.0 mcg	130	32.5 mcg
Pilchards (canned in tomato sauce)	14.0 mcg	215 (1 small can)	30.1 mcg
Herring	16.1 mcg	119	19.2 mcg
Salmon (canned in brine)	17.0 mcg	100	17.0 mcg
Trout	9.6 mcg	155	14.9 mcg
Mackerel	8.8 mcg	160	14.1 mcg
Sardines	12.3 mcg	86 (6 average)	10.6 mcg
Fresh Tuna	7.2 mcg	100	7.2 mcg
Salmon, grilled	7.1 mcg	100	7.1 mcg
Sun-dried shiitake mushrooms	45 mcg	10	4.5 mcg
Tuna (canned in brine)	3.6 mcg	100 (1 small can)	3.6 mcg
Fortified cereals	2.8–8.3 mcg	40	1.1–3.3 mcg
Eggs	1.8 mcg	75	1.4 mcg
Liver	1.1 mcg	100	1.1 mcg
Margarine	7.8 mcg	10	0.8 mcg
Vitamin E			
Sunflower seeds	49.5 mg	16 (1 tbsp)	8.0 mg
Almonds	24.2 mg	13 (6 whole)	3.1 mg
Hazelnuts	25.0 mg	10 (10 whole)	2.5 mg
Avocado	3.2 mg	75 (½ pear)	2.4 mg
Blackberries	2.37 mg	80	1.9 mg
Sunflower oil	49.2 mg	3 (1 tsp)	1.5 mg
Spinach	1.7 mg	90	1.5 mg
Peanuts	10.1 mg	13 (10 whole)	1.3 mg
Wheatgerm	22.0 mg	5 (1 tbsp)	1.1 mg
Brazil nuts	11.0 mg	10 (3 whole)	1.0 mg
Tomato	1.2 mg	85 (1 medium)	1.0 mg

Food component	amount per 100g	portion size (g)	amount per portion
Margarine	7.9 mg	10 (on one slice of bread)	0.8 mg
Eggs	1.1 mg	61 1 medium	0.7 mg
Canola oil	22.2 mg	3 (1 tsp)	0.7 mg
Mango	1.1 mg	40 (1 slice)	0.4 mg
Sesame seeds	2.5 mg	12 (1 tbsp)	0.3 mg
Olive oil	5.1 mg	3 (1 tsp)	0.2 mg
Fish and seafood omega-3 fatty acids			
Anchovies	1.400 mg	50 (1 small can)	700 mg
Mackerel	2500 mg	160	4000 mg
Trout	1300 mg	155	2015 mg
Swordfish	800 mg	140	1.120 mg
Cod	400 mg	120 (1 medium fillet)	480 mg
Herring	1700 mg	119	2023 mg
Salmon	1200 mg	100 (average steak)	1200 mg
Sardines (canned in sardine oil)	3.300 mg	100 (average can)	3.300 mg
Tuna	400 mg	100 (small can)	400 g
Selenium			
Brazil nuts (very variable content)	1530 mcg	12 (3 nuts)	153 mcg
Kidney	150 mcg	112	168 mcg
Lemon sole	60 mcg	170	102 mcg
Tuna (canned in oil)	90 mcg	92	83 mcg
Mackerel	30 mcg	160	48 mcg
Liver (lamb)	42 mcg	100	42 mcg
Sardines (canned)	41 mcg	100	41 mcg
Crab	37 mcg	85	32 mcg
Chicken	12 mcg	150	18 mcg
Turkey light meat	10 mcg	150	15 mcg
Shrimp	16 mcg	60	10 mcg
Egg	11 mcg	61	7 mcg

These figures are taken from McCance and Widdowson's "The Composition of Foods" and a number of scientific studies.

Appendix 4: References

Key references cited for each chapter. For a full list of all references please refer to www.surrey.ac.uk/diet-and-dementia

Introduction

Alzheimer's Research UK (2011) *Alzheimer's Research UK—Defeating Dementia*. Available at http://www.alzheimersresearchuk.org (accessed April 2014).

Alzheimer's Society (2014) *Alzheimer's Society—Leading the fight against dementia*. Available at http://www.alzheimers.org.uk (accessed April 2014).

Dementia UK (2014) *Dementia UK—Improving quality of life*. Available at https://www.dementiauk.org (accessed April 2014).

Antioxidants

Colombo. An update on vitamin E, tocopherol and tocotrienol-perspectives. *Molecules* 2010; 15(4): 2103–13.

Cordero et al. Vitamin E and risk of cardiovascular diseases: a review of epidemiologic and clinical trial studies. *Crit Rev Food Sci* 2010; 50(5): 420–40.

Devore et al. Dietary antioxidants and long-term risk of dementia. *Arch Neurol* 2010; 67(7): 819–25.

Harrison. A critical review of vitamin C for the prevention of age-related cognitive decline and Alzheimer's disease. *J Alzheimers Dis* 2012; 29(4): 711–26.

Luchsinger and Mayeux. Dietary factors and Alzheimer's disease. *Lancet Neurol* 2004; 3(10): 579–87.

Ricciarelli et al. Vitamin E and neurodegenerative diseases. *Mol Aspects Med* 2007; 28(5–6): 591–606.

Sayre et al. Oxidative stress and neurotoxicity. *Chem Res Toxicol* 2008; 21(1): 172–88.

Selenium

Akbaraly et al. Plasma selenium over time and cognitive decline in the elderly. *Epidemiology* 2007; 18: 52–8.

Berr C. et al. Cognitive decline is associated with systemic oxidative stress: the EVA study. Etude du Vieillissement Arteriel. *J Am Geriatr Soc* 2000; 48: 1285–91.

Burk R.F. et al. Selenoprotein P-expression, functions, and roles in mammals. *Biochim Biophys Acta* 2009; 1790: 1441–7.

Gao S. et al. Selenium level and cognitive function in rural elderly Chinese. *Am J Epidemiol* 2007; 165: 955–65.

Leszek J. et al. Colostrinin: a proline-rich polypeptide (PRP) complex isolated from ovine colostrum for treatment of Alzheimer's disease. A double-blind, placebo-controlled study. *Arch Immunol Ther Exp* (Warsz) 1999; 47(6): 377–85.

Olde Rikkert M. G. et al. Differences in Nutritional Status between very Mild Alzheimer's Disease Patients and Healthy Controls. *J Alzheimers Dis*

2014 Mar 10. [Epub ahead of print]

Perkins A.J. et al. Association of antioxidants with memory in a multi-ethnic elderly sample using the Third National Health and Nutrition Examination Survey. *Am J Epidemiol* 1999; 150(1): 37–44.

Rayman M. P. Selenium and human health. *Lancet* 2012; 379(9822): 1256–68.

Takemoto A.S. et al. Role of selenoprotein P in Alzheimer's disease. *Ethn Dis* 2010; 20(1 Suppl 1): S1-92-5.

Yim S.Y. et al. ERK activation induced by selenium treatment significantly down regulates beta/gamma-secretase activity and Tau phosphorylation in the transgenic rat overexpressing human selenoprotein M. *Int J Mol Med* 2009; 24(1): 91–6.

Polyphenols

Del Rio et al. Dietary (Poly)phenolics in human health: structures, bioavailability and evidence of protective effects against chronic diseases. A Comprehensive Invited Review. *Antioxi Red Signal* 2013; 18(14); 1818–92.

EFSA Panel on Dietetic Products, Nutrition and Allergies. Scientific Opinion on the substantiation of a health claim related to cocoa flavonols and maintenance of normal endothelium-dependent vasodilation pursuant to Article 13(5) of Regulation (EC) No 1924/20061. *EFSA Journal* 2012; 10(7): 2809.

Hooper et al. Effects of chocolate, cocoa, and flavan-3-ols on cardiovascular health:

a systematic review and meta-analysis of randomised trials. *Am J Clin Nutr* 2012; 95(3): 740–51.

Siervo *et al.* Inorganic Nitrate and Beetroot Juice Supplementation Reduces Blood Pressure in Adults: A Systematic Review and Meta-Analysis. *J Nutr* 2013; 143(6): 818–26.

Vitamin B

Dangour A. D. *et al.* B vitamins and fatty acids in the prevention and treatment of Alzheimer's disease and dementia: a systematic review. *J Alzheimers Dis*. 2010; 22(1): 205–24.

Douaud *et al.* Preventing Alzheimer's disease-related gray matter atrophy by B-vitamin treatment, *Proc Natl Acad Sci U S A* 2013; 110(23): 9523–28.

Lopes da Silva *et al.* Plasma nutrient status of patients with Alzheimer's disease: Systematic review and meta-analysis. *Alzheimers Dement* 2014; 10: 485-502.

Smith A. D. *et al.* Homocysteine-lowering by B vitamins slows the rate of accelerated brain atrophy in mild cognitive impairment: a randomised controlled trial. *PLoS One* 2010; 5(9): e12244.

Smith A. D. The worldwide challenge of the dementias: A role for B vitamins and homocysteine? *Food Nutr Bull* 2008; 29(2): S143–S172.

Vitamin D

Afzal S. *et al.* Reduced 25-hydroxyvitamin D and risk of Alzheimer's disease and vascular dementia. *Alzheimer's & Dementia* 2013.

Annweiler C. *et al.* Low serum vitamin D concentrations in Alzheimer's disease: a systematic review and meta-analysis. *J Alzheimers Dis* 2013; 33(3): 659–74.

Balion C. *et al.* Vitamin D, cognition, and dementia: a systematic review and meta-

analysis. *Neurology* 2012; 79(13): 1397–405.

Brouwer-Brolsma E. *et al.* Associations of 25-hydroxyvitamin D with fasting glucose, fasting insulin, dementia and depression in European elderly: the SENECA study. *Eur J Nutr* 2013; 52(3): 917–25.

Brouwer-Brolsma E. *et al.* Serum 25-Hydroxyvitamin D Is Associated With Cognitive Executive Function in Dutch Prefrail and Frail Elderly: A Cross-Sectional Study Exploring the Associations of 25-Hydroxyvitamin D With Glucose Metabolism, Cognitive Performance and Depression. *J Amer Med Assoc* 2013; 14(11): 852–e9.

Etgen T. *et al.* Vitamin D deficiency, cognitive impairment and dementia: a systematic review and meta-analysis. *Dementia and geriatric cognitive disorders* 2012; 33(5): 297–305.

Holick M. F. *et al.* Endocrine Society Evaluation, treatment, and prevention of vitamin D deficiency: an Endocrine Society clinical practice guideline. *J Clin Endocrinol Metab* 2011; 96: 1911–30.

Hyppönen E, Power C. Hypovitaminosis D in British adults at age 45 y: Nationwide cohort study of dietary and lifestyle predictors. *Am J Clin Nutr* 2007; 13(3): 860–8.

IOM (Institute of Medicine). Dietary Reference Intakes for Calcium and Vitamin D. Committee to Review Dietary Reference Intakes for Calcium and Vitamin D. Washington DC: The National Academies Press 2011. Institute of Medicine.

Lanham-New S. A. *et al.* Proceedings of the Rank Forum on Vitamin D. *Br J Nutr.* 2011; 105(1): 144–56.

Macdonald H. M. *et al.* Sunlight and dietary contributions to the seasonal vitamin D status of cohorts of healthy postmenopausal women living at northerly latitudes: a major cause for concern? *Osteoporos Int.* 2011; 22: 2461–72.

Pearce S. & Cheetham D. Diagnosis and management of vitamin D deficiency. *BMJ* 2010; 340(11): 5664–6.

Rossom R. C. *et al.* Calcium and vitamin D supplementation and cognitive impairment in the women's health initiative. *J Am Geriatr Soc* 2012; 60(12): 2197–205.

van der Schaft J. *et al.* The association between vitamin D and cognition: a systematic review. *Ageing Res Rev* 2013; 12(4): 1013–23.

Fats and fish

Berr C. *et al.* Olive oil and cognition: results from the three-city study. *Dement Geriatr Cogn Disord* 2009; 28(4): 357–64.

Calder P. C. and Deckelbaum R. J. Harmful, harmless or helpful? The n-6 fatty acid debate goes on. *Curr Opin Clin Nutr Metab Care* 2011 Mar; 14(2): 113–4.

Eskilinen M. The Effects of Midlife Diet on Late-Life Cognition. An Epidemiological Approach. Publications of the University of East Finland. Dissertations in Health Sciences 2014. Available at http://epublications.uef.fi/pub/urn_isbn_978-952-61-1394-4/urn_isbn_978-952-61-1394-4.pdf

Grant W. B. Trends in diet and Alzheimer's disease during the nutrition transition in Japan and developing countries. *J Alzheimers Dis* 2014; 38(3): 611–20.

Loef M. and Walach H. The omega-6/omega-3 ratio and dementia or cognitive decline: a systematic review on human studies and biological evidence. *J Nutr Gerontol Geriatr* 2013; 32(1): 1–23.

Uauy R., Dangour A. D. Nutrition in brain development and ageing: role of essential fatty acids. *Nutr Rev* 2006; 64(5 Pt 2): S24–33; discussion S72–91.

Solfrizzi V. *et al.* Dietary fatty acids in dementia and predementia syndromes: epidemiological evidence and possible underlying mechanisms. *Ageing Res Rev* 2010; 9(2): 184–99.

Sydenham E. *et al.* Omega 3 fatty acid for the prevention of cognitive decline and dementia. Cochrane Database Syst Rev. 2012; 6:CD005379.

Weichselbaum, E. Fish in the diet: A review. *Nutr Bull*. 2013; 38(2):128–77.

Dietary patterns

Gu Y. *et al*. Food combination and Alzheimer disease risk: a protective diet. *Arch Neurol* 2010b; 67(6)L 699–706.

Jacobs *et al*. Food synergy: an operational concept for understanding nutrition, *Am J Clin Nutr* 2009; 89(5): 1543S–8S.

NIH (2012). *What is the DASH eating plan?* Available at www.nhlbi.nih.gov/health/health-topics/topics/dash/ (Accessed April 2014).

Ozawa *et al*. Dietary patterns and risk of dementia in an elderly Japanese population: the Hisayama Study. *Am J Clin Nutr*. 2013; 97(5): 1076–82.

Psaltopoulou T. *et al*. Mediterranean diet, stroke, cognitive impairment, and depression: A meta-analysis. *Ann Neurol*. 2013; 74(4): 580–91.

Sofi F. *et al*. Accruing evidence on benefits of adherence to the Mediterranean diet on health: an updated systematic review and meta-analysis. *Am J Clin Nutr* 2010; 92(5): 1189–96.

USDA (2013). *US Healthy Eating Index*. Available at www.cnpp.usda.gov/healthyeatingindex.htm. (Accessed April 2014).

Willett W. *et al*. Mediterranean diet pyramid: a cultural model for healthy eating. *Am J Clin Nutr* 1995; 61(6): 1402S–1406S

Alcohol

Kim J. *et al*. Alcohol and cognition in the elderly: a review. *Psychiatry Investig* 2012; 9(1): 8–16.

Panza F. *et al*. Alcohol drinking, cognitive functions in older age, predementia, and dementia syndromes. *J Alzheimers Dis* 2009; 17: 7–31.

Panza F. *et al*. Alcohol consumption in mild cognitive impairment and dementia: harmful or neuroprotective? *Int J Geriatric Psych* 2012; 27(12): 1218–38.

Piazza-Gardner A. K. *et al*. The impact of alcohol on Alzheimer's disease: a systematic review. *Aging Ment Health* 2013; 17(2): 133–46.

Appendix 1

Bherer L. *et al*. A Review of the Effects of Physical Activity and Exercise on Cognitive and Brain Functions in Older Adults. *J Aging Res* 2013; 2013: 657508.

Behrman S. and Ebmeier K. P. Can exercise prevent cognitive decline? *Practitioner* 2014; 258(1767): 17–21, 2–3.

Erickson K. I. *et al*. Physical activity and brain plasticity in late adulthood. *Dialogues Clin Neurosci* 2013; 15(1): 99–108.

Gomez-Pinilla F. and Hillman C. The influence of exercise on cognitive abilities. *Compr Physiol* 2013; 3(1): 403–28.

Gregory M. A. *et al*. Brain health and exercise in older adults. *Curr Sports Med Rep* 2013; 12(4): 256–71.

Nagamatsu L. S. *et al*. Resistance training promotes cognitive and functional brain plasticity in seniors with probable mild cognitive impairment. *Arch Intern Med* 2012; 172(8): 666–8.

Tolppanen A. M. *et al*. Leisure-time physical activity from mid- to late life, body mass index, and risk of dementia. *Alzheimers Dement* 2014; pii: S1552–5260(14)00034–X.

Appendix 2

John Wiley & Sons, Ltd (2014). *Cochrane systematic reviews*. Available at www.thecochranelibrary.com/view/0/index.html. (Accessed April 2014).

Petticrew M. *et al*. Evidence, hierarchies and typologies: horses for courses. *J Epidemiol Community Health* 2003; 57(7): 527–9.

Sackett D. L. *et al*. Evidence based medicine: what it is and what it isn't. *BMJ* 1996; 312:7023.

Wikimedia Foundation, Inc. (Dec 2013). *Hierarchy of evidence. Available at* http://en.wikipedia.org/wiki/Hierarchy_of_evidence. (Accessed April 2014).

Index

Acknowledgments

First and foremost, we would like to thank our funders, the Waterloo Foundation, for recognizing the potential impact of an evidence-based cookbook aimed at reducing the risk of dementia in our aging population and enabling us to produce it.

We would also like to thank our most helpful and patient editor, Tara O'Sullivan, for whom nothing was too much trouble, our home-economist and food stylist Annie Nichols, who has an amazing eye for how food should be presented, and our talented photographer, Will Heap.

Our grateful thanks go to celebrity chef, Gino D'Acampo for providing us with some wonderful recipes and to John Walter and David Hill, chefs at the University of Surrey's Lakeside Restaurant, who searched their repertoire for dishes to fulfil our rigorous criteria.

We also acknowledge the contribution of Sophie Bruno who, as part of her final year Nutrition degree project at the University of Surrey, contributed to an early prototype version of this book.

We are very happy that Professor David Smith agreed to write the Foreword for our book; Prof. Smith's elegant work on the B vitamins and dementia has been an inspiration to us and others in this field.

Last but not least, we would like to thank our friends and families who both provided recipes, cooked them, and supported and encouraged us throughout this very demanding project.